RED-PILLING
IN A
CLOWN WORLD

CHARLES FOXTROT

Fisher King Publishing

RED-PILLING IN A CLOWN WORLD

Published by Fisher King Publishing
fisherkingpublishing.co.uk

Cover cartoon courtesy of the legend that is Bob Moran

Contents

1. Darren

"Darren - has - gone — COMPLETELY - FUCKING - MAD," I reported back to my wife in an urgently made phone call.

I was in southern Portugal, where we used to live. It was a stunning spring day, with completely blue skies, birds singing and a crystal-clear clarity of colours - as it always was. I was with my young daughter about to meet my old neighbour and drinking buddy for a coffee and a catchup. I had all my digs about Chelsea ready, and a few funnies saved up over the three years since we came back to the UK, I knew he would also be tooled up, and was expecting our usual banter where neither of us listened as we were always too keen to get our 'gem of a put down' out. We hadn't communicated much since then, so I was really looking forward to seeing his cheeky - son of East-End cockney jailbird, as he was, grin.

Waiting by the statue near the river, I was scanning up and down the cobbled streets for his unmissable gait.

What happened next made my brain feel like a Jackson Pollock.

A screech of shoddy brakes on his battered blue Ford Fiesta was quickly followed by, "Quick, get in," and a face with psychotic eyes, checking front, sides, and rear, as if a big, black-windowed gangster car was hot on his heels.

"Where're we going you knob-head"? I said through a laugh, "Can't you just park up, let's go for a coffee," I didn't really want to bundle my 6-year-old into the back of a soon-to-be bullet-peppered hatchback.

"No - mate, get in, it's important," he said — so, irresponsibly, we did, and sure enough he sped off like Mr Big was closing in.

"They are going to kill us, and your children mate," he said. Not quite the 'Liverpool are shite again', I was expecting!

What followed was a badly driven drive around the same circuit, several times, with him just barking words at me in a maniacal, urgent barrage. He didn't draw breath and all I could muster was a few "eh's," and "what's," before telling him to stop as a 6-year-old girl was sat behind us – "Stop man, let us out, I'll ring you later, honest."

Some of the things he was saying included names, organisations, and concepts I had heard of, but never really investigated, others seemed from ancient times, fantasy, or biblical.

Either way, he had obviously smoked too much hydroponic weed and was having a psychotic episode.

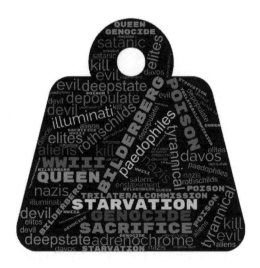

Darren's heavy weight he was offloading – Thanks mate (hope you get treatment)!

My final words to him were something like 'Great to see you enjoy research mate, why not do something useful like an open university degree?'

That was spring 2017.

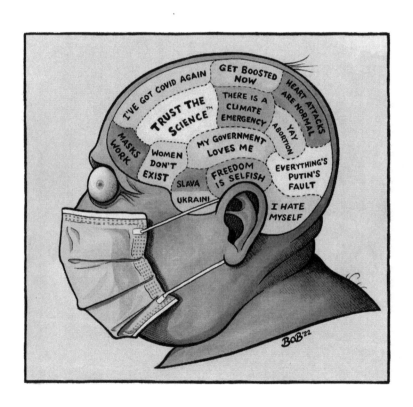

2. Introduction

Judging by my watch, it's five minutes to WWIII.

Hopefully, this book will still be read by someone, somewhere. It would have either aged very well or embarrassingly badly.

It is my personal experience of the last three years, living in a Clown World.

I am writing, essentially, a study in human behaviour – psychology - basic stuff, Pavlov's dogs' level. How humans react to a stimulus, creating behaviours, the avoidance of actions, and what you 'think you think'- Stimuli include the following:

Other People's Behaviour: friends, social media influencers, rock stars, sports stars, parents, social 'norms', the 'done thing', and etiquette. As an example, a random group of people pointing up at something in the sky or running away from something you can't yet see – the general reaction is to look up or run away also, maybe ask questions after, although it seems, maybe not so for everyone.

Visual images: Danger signs, TV adverts, News Stories, Public Service Announcements, Rules, Social Suggestions -or are they orders? e.g., 'Be Kind'- I am seeing that too much right now, 'Be Kind!' like you never thought about being so. 'Be Kind, or the Puppy gets it...' On that note, I have just read that the Labour Party in the UK is suggesting prison for calling a man in a dress, a man!

Basic Fears: Not just the risk of harm if you ignore the stimuli, but the risk of social exclusion if you go against the group. This could be just admitting to a guilty pleasure such as proudly owning the full ABBA back catalogue to your male bricklaying colleagues or something with more extreme consequences, like posting images of a Nazi AZOF brigade, doing their Blue and Yellow 'Sieg Heil' on LinkedIn. There may be great urges to do so, it feels like the right thing to do, but it would be a career suicide.

I have a great friend who 'awoke' at the same time as me, in fact, we had a mutual and sudden realisation together that something very bad was taking place, it made the hairs on the back of my neck prick up. I recall we were discussing the (fraudulent) PCR tests and the obviously staged case numbers, this could only mean one thing – a deliberate and coordinated attack on the People by our Government and many others around the world. It was like the moment I remember seeing a grainy black and white, haunted, J. Robert Oppenheimer's 'what have I done' moment, realising he had become "Death, the Destroyer of Worlds." Anyway, my friend has many corporate meetings and events every week where he is surrounded by fat cat CEOs, all staunch supporters of the latest booster, yet their own health has deteriorated rapidly, he simply can't say anything, in fact, he's been told not to say anything by the few colleagues who hide his little secret, as it would be the end of any deal currently being thrashed out and him financially ruined – I was going to say I don't know how he does it, how he bites his lip, but I guess I answered my question.

'Following The Herd' stems back to a 'safety in numbers' approach to survival, making sure you don't get separated and picked off by the predator, or at best – not to look stupid! Nobody wants either consequence, and it takes a very brave, or stubborn, person to do so intentionally. My Mother has always said to me 'Why can't you be like everyone else, just be normal'.

A great example is the Social Experiment conducted by 'Brain Games' on National Geographic. They filled a doctor's waiting room with actors and had them all sitting patiently waiting to be called for their appointment. A lady who was completely unaware of the experiment enters and takes her seat. A short while later a beep sounds, and all the actors stand up for a few seconds before sitting again. She looks bemused. A second beep sounds, and all the actors stand again; nothing is said but she looks around in confusion. On the third beep, everyone stands, including her, the subject, they sit again, and nothing is said. Sheep.

There must be something within those who are Awake, and actively making it known, that enables us to step outside of the herd. I know that I wouldn't have stood in the waiting room when a bell sounded, likewise, I just wouldn't wear a mask when waiting to collect my daughter outside her primary school – just me amongst a hundred masked sheep – just couldn't do it. There are hundreds of thousands of us – we all seem to share similar backgrounds that I will go into later, all seem to have been a little rebellious growing up, black sheep of the family, etc. Of course, the Normies will use that against us, 'Yeah, he was always a bit weird', the trouble, there, is that a lot of us are doctors, scientists, very well-educated and intelligent people, previously holding well-respected positions in society – we didn't all collectively go mad, yet some still argue that we did!

Social media, along with the mainstream media are very heavy influencers, TVs are always on, everywhere, even in places of leisure such as pubs or travel waiting areas and doctors' surgeries. If not the TV, it will be the radio and, if neither of those, Hollywood,

Computer Games, Sporting Events; and then we are all conditioned to whip our devices out every 10 minutes, you are subjected to a never-ending stream of 'News', Information, Misinformation, Disinformation – maybe Malinformation works as a better term – and Propaganda. A random glance as I write: It's a large rally for Palestinian freedom, I see a man with a megaphone on a stage, shouting, and in reply the crowd go -YAY!, "Palestine Justice!" – YAY!, "Gender Justice" – YAY!, "Climate Justice," - YAY! Really??? Yup, really.

It's a consistent bash on the head, drumming in the same messages and, in recent years, much scarier, fear-provoking, negative, and urgent, pointing us towards impending doom, and there are victims of hate everywhere, haters are rife, victims are OFFENDED for Christ's sake! They all say the same things and they all dictate the latest campaign we must all support and champion – remembering to be 'Kind', to be 'Responsible', to not kill your Grannies! And to think correctly. You mustn't think outside of the official box. If you do, somehow, you have gone from a reasonably middle ground, kind of 'mean no harm', 'salt of the earth', neighbour – to an evil racist. Seek help, repent, deprogram, exorcize your demons.

The problems all seem to be global now, global warming, global pandemics, global financial crash, requiring a global response – hmm, funny that.

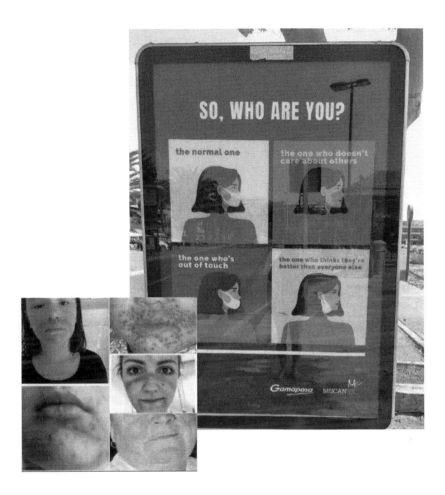

...the one with the bacterial respiratory infection?

This used to appear benign, yes, a bit lefty, increasingly woke, but seemingly harmless. Trump started to call them Fake News, and most of us may have laughed, for a while.

Then, for a lot of us, it became worrying, they were clearly lying, they were not reporting certain newsworthy stories – as an example the, what should have been historic, Abraham Accords in late 2020. These peace deals on Arab/Israeli relations were a stunning breakthrough mediated by the Trump administration (currently they are at full-blown war). There was barely a mention, if at all (they were clearly concentrating on building bad PR only, about staged riots in the blue states, due to the upcoming elections) - they were using the same sentences, in unison, as if all running from a script. They were creating the problem, and the solution came along instantly- which was always a net loss of freedom. 'Normies' lapped it up and encouraged such nuisances, grateful that their governments had planned for the greater good. Stockholm Syndrome. When the Nazis were exterminating the Jews in the 1940s, some of the victims were so much like our 'Normies', they would be thanking the trooper helping them up into the carriages to Auschwitz.

The Mainstream and social media, we later found out, thanks to Elon Musk, have been 'Social Engineering' for decades. Manipulating thought and beliefs, moulding a compliant groupthink, weakening the power of the people, and tampering with elections.

This book is about how a large section of society became 'AWAKE', I never liked the term, but it is difficult to think of another that describes those who realised they were being lied to and that an agenda was in play, a nefarious agenda and the key players were not only on TV, but amongst us.

Urgent action was required.

The problem for all of us is that we see the people around us, family, friends, and work colleagues just carry on as if everything was normal. The struggle to live in what we term a 'Clown World' is beyond bizarre. Most of us have a never-ending energy buzzing around us that stems from immense frustration. Not only do we have a knowledge of nefarious agendas threatening the very existence of our children, but we are also surrounded by people completely oblivious to it. It almost hurts – in fact, it does.

This book explores the personal experience of what we might call, waking up the Sheep, Red-pilling the Zombies, and Shaking up the Normies with Truth Bombs – whatever it is, it's the hardest thing any of us have ever attempted - ever. We receive abuse, ridicule, insults, and palpable hate, we lose friends and family and jobs. Of course, we are also known as Tin Foil Hat Wearers, Flat-Earthers, Whackjobs, Nutters, and the CIA's favourite, Conspiracy Theorists.

I have completely lost my best friend of 30 years, we were so alike, and I am gobsmacked at he has fallen hook, line, and sinker to the propaganda – he may say the same that I have fallen for the 'conspiracy theories' – when I started to express my concerns, he would say 'here you go, all conspiracy mental again'. We don't talk at all now, can't – the Elephant between us in the room is so massive that we both get firmly squashed against opposing walls.

It has been pointed out to me that calling the other side, 'Normies', or 'Leftists', is just playing into the hands of the real bad guys, the Cabal, who orchestrated this attack on humanity, it merely deepens the divide, I will try and temper the urge – Maybe 'Conspiracy Deniers'?

Some of us- not me (unless this book is very successful), who have large audiences, find they are suddenly accused of rape from decades ago – (hope my book isn't successful). Probably the one thing that can't be proven but guilt still sticks after the front-page trial by the corrupt media. We are fighting a real 'world war', an 'information war', one that boils down to good versus evil, freedom versus tyranny, life versus death, or servitude.

'The pen is mightier than the sword', often said but first by playwright Edward Bulwer-Lytton in 1839, is truer now than ever, we are fighting an information war that is not quite yet kinetic (at the time of writing) – there is a massive army around the world of keyboard warriors trying to defeat the evil 'Cabal' who own mainstream media – we are digital soldiers, whether we understand Q's version or not (more to come on that).

I will explain my personal journey to a sudden awakening from 2020 and the activities that followed. and include several accounts, with mind-blowing exchanges, of attempts to stir my brother, son, and Mother from their obvious slumbers, (published on Substack, throughout 2022 to Oct 2023). To give some balance, I invited my brother to give his take on my experiences with him throughout this period – unsure if this will materialise though. The Substacks were written live, while in a deep state of discombobulation, so they may sound emotionally charged.

In later chapters I pick out key events as they were unfurling, at a rapid pace, further cementing the terrible actions and plans of the deep-state players. Many reminders come from a Telegram Channel I set up designed specifically to capture a chronological record of these darkest, yet amazing and, IMHO, biblical times. Terrible, evil actions that most people around us still have no idea, in fact, a lot of them do not want to know, and some of them even think they are honest deeds from good people, 'because science doesn't lie', 'Bill Gates is kindly being philanthropic with his wealth' – such is their Cognitive Dissonance (a term that crops up a lot).

Along the way, week by week, we built up a great collection of artworks produced by clever unknown digital warriors hidden amongst us to encapsulate powerful messages for the time, 'a picture paints a thousand words' and that is how Memes became such an effective weapon for us. These people deserve so much praise and recognition, yet they do not seek it. Their effectiveness became even more apparent when we learned of the systemic censoring within the social media platforms, the ones we had naively thought helped us freely communicate – what a con that was. Bots and Algorithms picked up words the bad guys didn't want to spread and quietly hid them deep down in the unread gutters, but pictures slipped through - they make beautiful, thought-provoking, and effective truth bombs – and fit nicely on stickers!

Looking back only two years reveals a sinister time of coercion, lies, threats, and propaganda reaching deeper than any dystopian world imaginable, a bombardment. Looking at the images of state-sponsored fear porn and 'health advice' now leaves you in utter disbelief. Boy, did they want everyone jabbed, masked, and scared – some are pure comedy. It seems laughable until, like me, you lose a friend – in her thirties; Booster - swollen red legs - sepsis-leukaemia – dead, in only a few months.

Not only did it come from the 'Authorities', but friends and family turned into wild irrational shouty versions of their former selves, the vitriol quickly following fluffy pink virtue signalling is something to behold when looking back – hilarious. In fact, while researching and collating material from this period, it truly is from a 'Clown World', the book itself may happily reside on the comedy shelves.

There are various forms and degrees of 'Awakeness', and likewise, there are varying levels of Unconsciousness yet there is a huge divide between the two. It's a bit like being a little bit pregnant. You are either awake and cannot unsee what you see, or you are in a state of ignorance/denial/stupidity, etc.

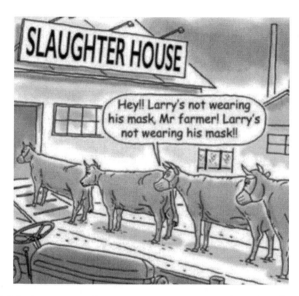

The divide between the two camps is very deep and very wide.

I am writing this as a battered, burnt-out, obviously awake bloke, who never chose this as a pastime. None of us would have chosen to do what we have been doing for the last 3 years, we hate it, it is hell.

So, I'm also angry, frustrated, and feel betrayed – forgive me if I am a little frosty with the dormant. I have calmed down significantly of late but it's fair to say that I've had my moments of despising them - traitors, collaborators, brainwashed zombies, turkeys voting for Christmas and dragging us all along to the slaughterhouse with them. However, there are hundreds of thousands of us who are very active. I know we have already been highly successful; I know that all children would have been injected if there wasn't an active resistance and, in that sense, we can feel some accomplishment. I also know we will win, more to the point, the battle has already been won and we are just playing out the final moves – more on that to come later.

Today's insistence on the virtues of *diversity* creates *division*, some of us *know* that is by design, some *think* an (over) eagerness to follow a vision of harmony, either way – it divides. The divisions between the sexes, politics, race, culture, and gender do not seem as wide as the gap between the Awake and the Not.

My experience is that both sides are firmly entrenched at the time of writing. My side, the Awake has grown tired and exasperated with the other side, most have worn themselves out trying to shake them up and the other side seems to just resort to patronising insults. It is so polarising, yet there is only one truth – one side is in for one hell of a surprise!

I believe there are four classifications of 'Normies'. 'Normie', I believe, is the best and most apt name for them, it reflects their modus operandi. I am not including any of the active deep state players here, some of those are very close to us in Local Government, Education, The Police, Hospitals, and perhaps neighbours. We don't know who or where, exactly, as this 'Black Hat' plan installed the base of the tyranny pyramid over decades. It was communism by stealth. They are either corrupt or controlled, or they have a 'kompromat' to keep hidden.

Just to index, – the active baddies and their masters are referred to as; The Cabal, The Khazarian Mafia, The Elite, The Illuminati, The Deep State, The Black Hats, and maybe, Bastards.

Normie classifications

1. Normies with no idea or inclination. These people are stupid. They were surely bred as cannon fodder. Pastry, vapes & dumb-down TV. 'Yeah, that's fucking right mate'- they say to whatever. 'My body, My choice' AND 'Vax Mandates -Yay!'.
2. Normies who watch mainstream media, hear whisperings of things being a bit off, but keep their blinkers fully forward set. Argue back but with Google answers or, if shooting from the hip, they are strongly-wrongly opinionated. Hatefully accuse us of 'HATE'. Ukraine & Rainbow flags and Masked bio pics. Gaslighters. More cannon fodder but with nicer boots.
3. Normies who know, have seen some evidence, but wish they hadn't and walk around with their fingers in their ears going 'La La La La La'. They just shout insults. The science is settled, no debate. Collaborators.
4. The fourth covers people who know we are under attack from tyrants but do nothing about it, assuming somehow it will just right itself. Act normal and it will go away. Selfish and Cowardly.

Selfish and Cowardly is a very strong accusation, especially if levelled at close family (probably not the best tactic), but that is what it boils down to.

I say selfish because there is no urgency or real intention to do anything that may help save the futures of ALL children, yes, they are doing everything they can to build a great life for their immediate families, protecting their families no doubt, but this isn't enough to save the next generation. It certainly won't put a dent into the advancement of the enemy.

I say cowardly because, if they know me, they see how people think I am mental, or how people shy away from talking with me or how I have lost friends and business opportunities by being vocal – they don't want that. Maybe they just see how I have aged 10 years in 3! They are in social circles that are firmly manipulated into the masked character in the cartoon by 'Bob', with the brain compartments – they tick all the boxes. You start to question one and you will be labelled a Far Right, Racist Homophobe, Climate Denier, Putin lover, and Anti-Vaxer. They don't want that. You will find that most people who are non-awake tend to believe the whole set and most awake expose the whole set – both sides tend to be all-in.

I use that cartoon daily on Twitter, now 'X' – if I am arguing against anyone about Ukraine, Vaccine Damage, Trans rights, The Climate Crisis, etc – and they resort to insults, I just send the pic saying 'This is you, isn't it' – they never respond! Such a powerful weapon.

'The Awake' – classifications.

1. One step on from the fourth Normie. Aware and questioning. Questioning openly amongst their peers.

2. Awake and a 'Truther'- This term always entertained me as it is widely used but it implies the holder of such a title dictates what is true. As in Animal Farm, some Truthers are more Truthier than others. Active and vocal. Attend marches and outreach events. Active in Truther Channels. Heroes. Tired, very tired.

3. Awake and addicted to 'Hopium' – a term used by some Truthers to denigrate people like me who understand and talk about things like Q, 'The Plan', Trump, and Devolution – all to be explained in a later chapter. Very active, some are 'Anons,' helping to decode evidence of 'the plan' and often attempting to help Truthers feel there is a 'White Hat' plan playing out as designed to keep them from despair. Exhausted.

4. Awake, often well-known, celebrities, top medics, scientists, journalists, and politicians bravely sticking their heads above the parapet – often getting shot. Superhuman.

Infighting amongst the Awake is and has been a great problem, of course the deep-state players welcome this, we often play right into their hands. Truthers often label us on the Q side, 'Qtards', Hopium fools, and suckers for falling for a 'Psyop' designed for us just to sit back and wait to be saved while we burn. Of course, none of us just sat back, we were all, and still are very active. Yes, maybe there is a big double psyop in play, accepted as a possibility, but you will read in the final few chapters why I think not.

Then there are the 'Shill Callers', I have defended many brave souls, giving everything to help the cause. Defended so much that

I have been kicked off some channels for being a troublemaker. In my view, their net actions are paramount, look at the message not the messenger. Yet there are people in the 'Awake' channels deciding they are 'shills' due to some old photo or apparent connection. 'Shill', they declare, and, bang, everything they say and do loses credibility. This is the Awake doing the Cabals work for them – in fact some of the 'Shill Callers' are probable infiltrators -controlled opposition - installed to do just that, they are shills calling out shills – although, unfortunately, most 'Shill Callers' just seem to lack intelligence. Their reasoning is less apparent to me than their pack mentality.

The survey

It feels that people are waking up, at least that's what I hear. Surely people can see the vax injuries, the unwell zombies, the brain fogged. Surely, they can see through the propaganda. Well, I really am not so sure. I think we are stuck, stale mate, 'us and them'. There was only one way to find out, I reasoned, and that was to go out there and ask. What do people think? If they are asleep, what type are they and if awake, how strong?

I thought the best way would be to simply show a series of images and ask for their gut reaction – good or bad. Good person/ bad person, good idea/bad idea, good policy/bad policy, agree/ disagree etc. No discussion a simple binary answer, if possible.

So, the images.

1.   A syringe and a vial of Covid-19 vaccine
2.   A person in lockdown wearing a mask

3. Carbon Net Zero
4. Joe Biden
5. Donald Trump
6. WEF/Klaus Schwab
7. WHO/Tedros Ghebreyesus
8. The fullest LGBTQ++++++ flag
9. Ukraine/Zelensky
10. BBC News
11. Quote, 'The right to free speech is more important than the content of the speech'
12. Bill Gates

I bought a clipboard to look 'legit' and 'knocked-up' a tick chart. Clipping my phone horizontally on the board allowed me to scroll through the images while ticking the sheet underneath. One of my wife's great ideas – otherwise I was needing three hands (something I talk about later on).

Firstly, I have to say, I didn't enjoy the experience. Most people hate the sight of some gimp approaching with a clipboard and a silly smile. Also, I really didn't fancy engaging with most of them. I had to though, I had to get a real 'as they come' sample.

I only engaged with 20 but felt that was enough. Most participants wanted discussion some started to change their minds as they contemplated further, of course, this was banned!

The results

1. A syringe and a vial of Covid-19 vaccine – Good 12 Bad 8
2. A person in lockdown wearing a mask – Good 8 Bad 12

3. Carbon Net Zero – Good 14 Bad 6
4. Joe Biden – Good 5 Bad 15
5. Donald Trump – Good 1 Bad 19
6. WEF/Klaus Schwab – Good 12 Bad 8
7. WHO/Tedros Ghebreyesus – Good 13 Bad 7
8. The fullest LGBTQ++++++ flag – Good 16 Bad 4
9. Ukraine/Zelensky – Good 18 Bad 2
10. BBC News – Good 13 Bad 7
11. Quote, 'The right to free speech is more important than the content of the speech' – Good 8 Bad 16
12. Bill Gates – Good 15 Bad 5

Some interesting points

Everyone entered into a 'discussion' despite me not wanting to.

All of those (bar two) who gave a 'bad' answer, regarding the jabs, said they had taken the first two, and maybe a booster or two but won't take anymore.

Many of those against masks and lockdowns went on to say they would comply if they were asked to in the future, so I think the 'good' answers were higher in a practical sense.

Most people said bad regarding Biden because they felt he was too old and had some health issues, three followed their answer with 'better than the one they had before'.

Everyone hated Trump, except one guy and he was Canadian. The Canadian was the only person who was completely and enthusiastically wide awake, a few others were obviously well on their way.

Most people did not recognise the face of Klaus Schwab and

most people didn't really know who the WEF were, or what they did so could not give informed answers. (I take the fact that a large percentage did not know who Schwab was, as a clear sign of mass 'asleep-ness' – how can it be that people don't know who this raving 'James Bond Villian' psychopath is?? How?? It's beyond me.)

People saying 'good' to the WHO didn't all know who Tedros was.

Those against the full LGBTQ++++ flag couldn't actually say 'bad' but they would give a 'look'. Obviously, they have been trained to think they were morally wrong to think that. Ditto Ukraine.

A lot of those saying 'Good' to the BBC, followed up with 'generally', so I detected an element of distrust.

People have obviously been swayed against the fundamental right to free speech, 'Hate Speech' and 'blablaphobia' seem to have got into their vocabulary.

And Bill Gates just wants to help humanity bless him.

My conclusion is that most people out there, by a long way, are still as asleep as they were almost 4 years ago. Conditioned.

3. Hold on a minute...

Feb 2020

"Shit, Shit, Shit, Shiiiiiiiit! Quick, go and ask Mum which gym she used last night." I waited nervously for my daughter to return, and the reply was bad, very bad.

It was the very same one used by the bloody SUPERSPREADER!! Same day, same gym, they tracked his movements. He was the Bubonic version of a Michelin restaurant inspector; you don't know they've been until they're gone. Like the mark of Zorro, but scary, very scary, his calling card was instant death. We knew it because we had seen them on the news in China. One minute standing happily waiting for a bus, the next, a little wobble, then splat, face down dead like a collateral skittle.

We had also seen them in Italy, hundreds of ambulances descending on a small-town hospital, corridors full of pre-death people wheezing into face tubes, wide eyes petrified behind windowed oxygen helmets. The Superspreader had picked up his contagion in Singapore before flying near there. French Alps, in some ski resort before flying directly to us, our gym and local pub. How was I going to tell my wife she is due to drop dead? Shit - that means all of us. Doomed.

At that time nobody knew who the Superspreader was, was he a bird, was he a plane? All we knew was he lurked amongst us. If he hadn't got us the first time, it will come – the virus survives on steel and plastic for hours(!) so they say, how much steel and plastic does the gym have for fuck's sake?? Clearly, we are stuck right in the epicentre of the mother of pandemics. I had to prepare while being so thankful of those brilliant scientists at the World Economic Forum and the World Health Organisation who had foreseen the potential the year before and had planned our safe route out (for those who survived). They were one step ahead, they even had tests ready to go. Amazingly, they had set up a multi-national dry run to test a pre-planned coordinated response for such an event just the year before. Visionaries.

And it was spreading around the world, quickly. We saw very similar pictures coming out of Brazil – uncanny how similar they were, obviously, they shared the same architectural preferences, ambulance designs, and uniforms. Latin cousins.

The numbers of cases in the UK were nearly hitting the tens – eight in fact!! Sky News built a special daily death stats board obviously cribbed from their cricket department. The BBC had their version and we watched daily, then hourly. The numbers were growing. China reported 44,276 cases with 1,110 dropping dead. 'Superspreader' had been responsible for 11 cases so far, infecting them in France, and of those, five were now in the UK, five in France, and one in Majorca -God help the world! It was very early days but, clearly, he had pre-killed the whole bloody town.

OK – be positive for the kids, maybe we got lucky so far, time for urgent action. Let's do this.

Do I lock my wife away upstairs in quarantine? Build an airlock to place food and water?

Within days the daily scores were rising, and we had reports coming in from around the world, all rising. A bit like the second half of the Eurovision Song Contest we went from one country to another with their scores, England was less, as usual – but it was here and each day it was spreading. There was talk of quarantine camps in China. Gulags, but nice ones. Nevertheless, this was our looming fate.

I took to gargling whiskey and tee tree oil steam breathing, towel over the head, face in a bowl, the hotter the better – it was intuitive and made total sense.

The Nurses and Doctors were, we assumed, flat-out exhausted, sifting through the dead and almost dead, desperate for Ventilators, (poor Matt Hancock, our unassuming and honest baby-faced Health Secretary, was pleading for them on TV, in tears, if only I had a few to spare, but no, I was useless). The good news was that James Dyson, our brilliant modern-day Barnes Wallis had turned his vacuums into ventilators in just 10 days! I presume a simple suck-to-blow job.

The nurses were defiantly carrying on while colleagues were dropping – they were absolute heroes. We all clapped and banged our pots and pans, in our road we even had glasses of wine in hand to share a drink whilst poking our heads out of the windows and the doors, I imagined Spitfires growling into action high above. Somehow, they found the time to also raise our spirits with wonderfully choreographed dances, becoming ever complex, it became an inter-hospital, international TikTok competition. We were great, but I thought the Australians were slightly ahead, having first-mover advantage.

How, will it get inside our house? Of course, Food! From the supermarkets, hundreds of grubby, viral hands picking up produce and putting them down again for me to buy and bring home. We gotta eat – what can I do?

I had read that pure alcohol kills Covid, actually, not pure as that evaporates too quickly, 70% was best. Amazon delivered 20 bottles and a decent sprayer within days, I figured that would last me a month, so already had a follow-up order in place.

I ordered everyone to stay in, I would be the brave one to hit the shops, grab our needs quickly, exit smoothly, and return to base with a precision of execution. The dangerous bananas, cauliflowers, packs of mince and toothpaste etc were all placed into a plastic laundry bin to the left of the downstairs sink, an empty and fully sprayed one ready to the right. One by one, each product was passed from left to right via the sink where they were sprayed and rotated, sprayed, and rotated horizontally, spayed and rotated vertically, my rubber-gloved hands developed the perfect technique.

I even sprayed the sprayer – point upwards, spray a few times, and twirl it up through the mist – and then soon adding the 'backward flip throw and catch' (single-hander) to eliminate the gloved hand contact flaw. 100% Sterile. I imagined that I would end up teaching others pretty soon, noticing how some long-haired beardy chap called Joe was raking it in with his fitness at home for kids' programs, everyone was doing it in their pyjamas. Soon, everyone will be doing the backward flip throw and catch in their PJ's. Everyone was learning the new normal. That great British wartime spirit had returned. All in it together. Happily.

This was how we survived, for two weeks, we were neither ill, nor dead. The case numbers were rocketing, 'get tested, get tested' the TV would say, everyone needs to be tested. The morning briefings now involved the Prime Minister and the top

Government Scientists and Medical Officers, we had the Vallance, Whitty, and Van-Tam daily show – I almost called it a 'puppet show' but of course, this was deadly serious - we were all in deep trouble. Get Tested!

Then Boris was admitted to hospital, after clapping for heroes, his mild symptoms took a turn for the worse, reports came in that he was gravely ill. I liked him, he was a libertarian and he stood up to those radical left, the hysterical, crying, Anti-Brexit opposition – when there was an opposition – I liked him and I became very worried he wouldn't pull through, I even said a little prayer. He recovered but seemed a very different character after.

We were allowed out for an hour to exercise. Seemed logical. I ventured out bravely, had a run by the sea, slipping my mask slightly up to my upper lip occasionally, when away from others to get better inhalations. Incredibly, a sweaty runner swept past and coughed! Right next to me, coughed! No mask, killing me without a care. I was literally looking for Police, he needs to be stopped. I was livid, and probably infected.

On my way home, I was thinking how odd it was that I had yet to know someone who had keeled over or was even ill. I bumped into two doctor friends of mine, they were masked and worried but said they had not yet encountered any real worrying cases – loads of hypochondriacs but no, the wave was yet to hit – but we had the Superspreader, we were the UK's epicentre, strange.

Then I thought about the poor check-out staff in the big supermarkets, handling thousands of bananas, cauliflowers, packs of mince and toothpaste every day from hundreds of filthy, germ-ridden shoppers passing along their conveyor belt, every day –

they must be dropping like flies. How are these places even still open?

Hmmm, maybe I should go and find out.

Tesco's was nearest so I wandered up there with a plan, I would buy one small item, pass through the till, and have a friendly little chat with the employee. How are you? How is the store coping? You must have a lot of colleagues getting sick. I went through three checkouts – more of a journey than it sounds due to a strictly mapped out lane system for those going towards a checkout and those still shopping in alternate isles for footfall going North, and every other for South - and got the same response. 'Fine thanks', 'we're coping', 'think we must be lucky, don't know of anyone being sick yet'.

I made sure my chats were casual, 'off the cuff' chit-chats, wondering if they were being primed to say this, didn't want it looking like I was a reporter – presuming at this stage there were real reporters also digging for facts.

Hmmm, I then went to the big ASDA, the same answers, Sainsbury's, the same. The most exposed in our community are not getting sick, and that was before the Perspex barriers.

Hold on a minute... hold on... Holy Shit... Something isn't right... this really doesn't add up.

THIS – IS – A – FUCKING – CON

And that is how I woke up – a complete, unshakeable, and permanent 180-degree turn.

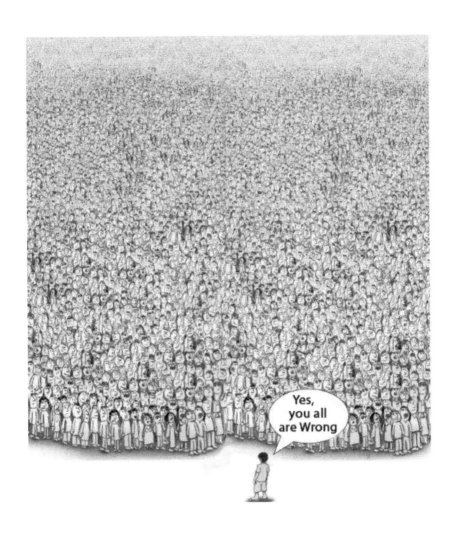

4. How to lose £4 Million

2019, what an awesome year. After eight years of trial and error, rebuilding, tweaking, adding, removing, and modifying, I had built my digital platform. It was a revolutionary disrupter for a massive market – Dragon's Den was calling. The show where you pitch your unique idea, the gap in the market where there is a market in the gap, in my mind they would all bid against each other for it and I'd end up with all five.

'Give me your figures for year one', one would say, 'er, well I've only just built it', I guess I would have replied. 'So, it's just a shiny concept, no proof of concept, just concept, prototype, beta...', they would say... yeah, in reality, it wouldn't go well.

So, I set up a company, built a simple website, attached the platform, and put out a few email ads to a few key players. Not sold one, no subscribers, no customers. Then a call from some wide boy, jolly but smart Londoner, I imagined a pinstripe suit, like a barrow-boy trader. 'This is what we want mate, come and see us tomorrow if you can, I'll ping you the address, midday, cheers bruvver'.

The next day, I walked into the Mayfair office and was led into the boardroom. They had a big screen set up and passed me the cable, 'Go on then, we're ready, plug this in your laptop and give us a demo'. About eight of them sat back and I just talked through what it did, how it worked, and what it will do with a few more tweaks.

Cut to the chase, two weeks later I had sold my company and my platform for ONE MILLION ENGLISH POUNDS. Well, it was a share roll-up, so shares in their company to that value. At the time they were listed in the top 60 fastest-growing companies in the UK, and they would be floating on the London Stock Exchange in 2021 with an expected 4 -10 X value. Congratulations, said the CEO, you're going to be a very wealthy man.

'Five bottles of those please', pointing to the £40 Champaign. Never done anything like that before, or since, nice feeling.

The AMG Mercedes company car was delivered the following week, just after I bought my BOSS watch, I had an office in Mayfair and an £80K job with a bunch of bonuses – and a golden hello.

That was it, job done, you finally made it. Made for life, never any more money worries, debts, or stress. That was all behind me and the family, the doubters had egg all over their faces, what joy.

Security for life! Gloat away son, gloat for England, boy you deserve it. Guaranteed - bar some 'Act of God' ☺☺☺!! You know, some kind of 'Force Majeure' ☺☺☺☺!!! Biblical Flood, Tsunami, Earthquake, you know, Pestilence, Pandemic... Oh, Wait, What?

It was March 2020, and we were going to present my creation to the whole market at the biggest industry show of the year at London's ExCel arena. All set to go, banners printed, suit dry cleaned, and then came the news. 'ExCel London to become the county's first Nightingale Hospital – Beds being delivered immediately'.

'Oh, and here's your Furlough letter, you will now receive 40% of your salary (from Rishi) and do not even attempt to contact us or enter your office – have a great day, stay safe'. [Stay Safe – they all started to say that, customer service employees, letters from banks – fuck off with your 'stay safe' – Stay Free more like!]

What followed was a tumble from the signs of success. First the car, then the house, then the sympathy. I found myself just walking up and down the beachside path, I even did a charity run that resulted in hip damage – just to compound things.

I was also 'Waking Up'- waking to the realisation that people wanted us dead, literally.

My actions turned to rebellion, and I bought a 'They're Lying to You' T-shirt for my public walks.

My Mayfair office seemed like a strange dream, a past life.

The months ahead are documented later, but fast forwarding to lockdowns. All other businesses that my employer company 'fed off', were also on furlough, they loved it, 90% pay and they could sit around on their arses. Naturally, that meant my new company had zero income, they called in the receivers and, 'Hey Presto', I lost all my shares – literally £ Millions. Everything gone. Back to square one, except this time we had a government hell-bent on destroying us.

Naturally, this was all my fault. So some thought. 'How did you let this happen?'

Later, my family seemed to rationalise my apparent mental illness by saying I was driven by the bitterness of losing everything. Ahh, that's why! They would say, poor him, he's been reduced to an 'angry with the world' victim. Too right I was angry with the world, them included but this certainly was not my driver, our children were.

In time I will get justice, and I will sue the government for illegal lockdowns. I know there will come a time. Yes, they are currently holding a Covid Inquiry, a lot of people are getting exposed for their incompetence, but this is a deep-state sham inquiry, 100% designed to ultimately conclude they didn't lock down hard, or fast enough. We know your game!

I will get justice but, for now, we fight.

5. The Staging of a CaseDemic

There are two major tactics used against us.

1. The one devised by Karl Marx where you accuse your enemy of doing something (bad) while, in actual fact, you are in the process of doing it yourself. It makes it so much harder for them to make accusations – it renders those accusations 'second-hand' and retaliatory. Gaslighting. A great example of this is the election cheating Hillary Clinton led Dems bleating on about 'having to save democracy' from the Jaws of Trump - gimme a break!

2. Allow your enemy to have information that is correct and incriminating for you but also give them a bunch of fake information mixed in, let them shout from the rooftops, let them expose what you are up to, but then release the evidence that the fake bits are fake. It will render them as baseless conspiracy theorists, unreliable, and paranoid. The real stuff simply gets mixed in and the whole thing is forever 'debunked', 'fact-checked', and hogwash nonsense.

Within days of knowing the 'pandemic' was at best highly suspicious and at worst a massive nefarious attack on the people, I, and thousands of others, set about a quest for some truth, some facts. We knew Google wouldn't help, we knew the mainstream media wouldn't offer anything, and we simply had to find safe platforms operating without censorship and 'Big Government' control.

Parler was that place, some very interesting material was also appearing on YouTube, but didn't always hang around for long. Parler was a social media platform that allowed access to like-minded individuals who had access to some seemingly reliable information from some seemingly reliable people - scientists and doctors among them.

Parler was soon taken down by the deep-state players, but then we found, Telegram, Signal, Rumble, and Gettr. We were growing rapidly in numbers and becoming better at sifting through the information, policing it ourselves, flagging disinformation. As best as we could.

The 'pandemic' was ramping up, case numbers spiralling, and nobody knew anyone who was sick.

A friend of mine, though, had an uncle who fell down some stairs, broke his pelvis, which released some fatty clots that travelled to his lungs and killed him. He was never ill previously and, although in a lot of pain going to hospital, he was otherwise not unwell. Two days later my friend was told he died of Covid. We were hearing of similar stories from all around the country, in fact, the world.

By the sea, where I lived, there is a very long and busy main road that covers a couple of miles running next to the promenade where most of the city walk – when not locked down. At weekends, when there was a large 'audience', it was becoming very noticeable that Ambulances with sirens and blue flashing lights were going east and west along the road almost every ten minutes. It was like the scene in 'The Blues Brothers', with the bedsit next to the trains, a 'joke' of frequency. There is a main hospital at one end so it seemed legitimate, but I thought I would investigate – I followed one, in my car. I actually sat with my rear backed into an alley and waited, like a traffic cop. Hearing the wailing, I inched forward to see one coming, I slipped out behind it. I followed it as much as I could, heading toward the hospital, we were getting close, but no, it turned the wrong way and headed down a smaller lane by the beach, turning its blue lights and sirens off at the junction. Normal cars were not allowed access, so I went around the roundabout and found myself behind another one, going the other way. Again, I followed but was getting further back until it was barely visible, but I did notice the flashing lights go off. Five minutes later I saw it parked up and one single occupant, the driver was entering a house cramming a sandwich in his mouth – certainly didn't look like he was attending an emergency. I took a photo and he looked at me as I did it. This looked, felt, and smelt staged.

I have no proof it was staged, and I am aware there is even an argument that if there were a deadly contagion spreading amongst us that people were not taking seriously, why not scare the pants off them (as Matt Hancock later said). Maybe that is a responsible tactic – like what parents do with 'stranger danger'.

The UK had its 'Nudge Unit' and SAGE, teams of 'experts' and behavioural scientists. We learned fairly early who made up these groups. One such character being Professor Niel Ferguson from the Imperial College, he was providing the government with projected deaths from his computer models, it was very high, and we were in deep trouble, he said. Previously, as later reported in The Spectator, he told us 200 million people will be killed by Bird Flu (it was 282, yes 282, no zeros after), 65,000 people will die in the UK from swine flu (it was 457 – he is getting better at it), foot and mouth disease in the UK required neighbouring farms killed their livestock - despite no evidence of infection (6 million animals were culled at a cost of £10 billion to the economy), around 50 - 150 thousand people will die from mad cow disease in the UK (it was 177). So, good form.

We soon found out that his covid-19 modelling was based on a 13-year-old computer code intended for use for an influenza pandemic, not coronavirus. His report projected 2.2 million deaths for the US. He obviously 'believed' his own predictions so strongly, as he later broke lockdown rules for a shag - twice.

So, daily cases by March 2020 were 6,338, by November it had reached 33,470 – daily (I still didn't know anyone who had it). I watched as bags of testing kits were being handed out like emergency bread at a disaster zone, people clambering to grab theirs – 'What are you doing? You do know you are going to cause lockdowns with this nonsense?' I shouted at them. 'It's utter nonsense, you lot are going mad and you're gonna drag us all down, you stupid, stupid people'. Just couldn't help myself but I knew they would lock down because of this, such an obvious tactic, it's what they want and then there will be suffering, real suffering - not knowing I would be one of the first, and in a major, several million pounds way. I think that was my first bit of public action -much more to come.

They were handing out 7 (why 7?) boxes of PCR test kits to everyone who passed just about any street corner – test, test, test, was the mantra. Funnily enough, the more they tested - the higher the number of 'Cases'. Go figure. Also, they had explained why nobody 'real' seemed to be ill - they were ASYMPTOMATIC, yes, dying of a dreadful Spanish Flu-like pandemic, but no symptoms. Ah, good one, I thought.

The RT-PCR GOLD STANDARD, 'our saviour', it picked up the virus from the asymptomatic and made them a 'case'. By then, of course, millions of poor scared people became convinced their seasonal runny nose was about to kill them. There were lots of customers.

Digging around the internet for information, we (a growing Parler tribe) became aware of the following information.

- Kary Mullis, a healthy surfing American Biochemist, was awarded the 1993 Nobel Prize in Chemistry for his creation of the PCR – Polymerase Chain Reaction - technique.
- He had many documented clashes with Dr Fauci and strong suspicions over the causes of AIDS.
- He died in 2019 – we thought conveniently.
- Allegedly, German Scientist, Christian Drosten had (very quickly) developed a version of PCR, called RT-PCR for use in Covid 19 viral detection. A review, by a consortium of scientists, into the scientific evidence backing the test -the 'Corman-Drosten Paper', produced serious concerns. They concluded; *"It was severely flawed with respect to its biomolecular and methodological design. A detailed scientific argumentation can be found in our review "External peer review of the RTPCR test to detect SARS-CoV2 reveals 10 major scientific flaws at the molecular and methodological level: consequences for false positive results," which we herewith submit for publication in Eurosurveillance. Further,*

the submission date and acceptance date of this paper are January 21st and January 22nd, respectively. Considering the severe errors in design and methodology of the RT-PCR test published by "Eurosurveillance," this raises the concern whether the paper was subjected to peer-review at all."

- Apparently, Jan 10-12th, 2020, the first sequences of the Sars-CoV2 virus were published. Jan 13th, (the next day!!), the WHO accepts Drosten's PCR as the Gold Standard. Jan 21st, The Corman–Drosten protocol paper was released. Jan 22nd (the next day!!) the peer review is complete. Incredibly, a Berlin manufacturer had fully functioning Drosten-developed PCR test kits ready for worldwide shipping on Jan 10th (same day as the first sequence!!). You may want to re-read that!
- Kary Mullis made it very clear that if you cycle the amplification too many times, you can pick up virtually anything, any fragment of any dead RNA. Anything over around 30 cycles would produce irrelevant results. PCR could NOT, he said, detect infectious virus.
- RT-PCR was being cycled up to 45 - to pick up disease in the asymptomatic, essential so they could keep ahead of the spread, they said.
- Tanzania's president revealed that a Goat, a Quail, and a Papaya had tested positive - things were getting ridiculous.

A reply to one of my FOI (Freedom of Information – an absolute Godsend for us 'truthers') requests revealed that our local hospital cycled at 40 and tested all inpatients every other day. Maybe that's how my friend's uncle ended up with 'Covid'? Not 'maybe'.

Later into 2021, (after the introduction of the jabs) they would turn the cycles down to 30 and make the tests a little harder to get, less frequently done. Strange as it may seem, the case numbers went down – 'see, the vaccines work', said the man on the Telly! Same man keeled over on Telly a few months later. Lol.

I wrote to my MP, a very senior Labour one. Pointed out everything wrong with the RT-PCR tests, explained how they will lead to unnecessary destruction, and how he can avoid getting himself incriminated by taking a stand – he couldn't say he didn't know. I received reams of official data back about how the tests were 'Gold Standard', 'Rigorously Tested', 'Peer Reviewed', 'Life Savers' – a typical 'the science is settled' response. We exchanged several emails leading up to a point where the MPs were due to vote on lockdown bills. My final email said this:

"While I wait for your response,

I must remind you that if you vote for a lockdown, you are doing it based on incorrect projections by SAGE which are based on the fraudulent use of PCR. You have enough evidence to know this. Lockdowns will cause far more harm than this virus that is not causing excess deaths.

If you vote for a lockdown, you will be making the biggest mistake of your career because it will ultimately end it.

There may well be court action for the biggest crime against humanity since the Nazis and parliament will be complicit.

A lot of us will be watching to see how people vote.

Good luck"

I didn't receive any further communication from him.

One would expect a pandemic to cause deaths, more deaths than usual. Call me cynical but I would have thought more deaths would mean more burials or cremations. A simple FOI to councils around the country showed, on average, there were no more burials or cremations in 2020 than the previous 10 years. Apparently, we had a slight flu epidemic in 2015 – who knew??

A few examples below suggest our pandemic was a bit of a rubbish one. Unless someone was hiding the bodies – I mean there were over 33,000 'cases' per day in November 2020!

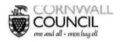

CORNWALL
COUNCIL
one and all · onen hag oll

Reference Number: 101005540478

Response provided under: Environmental Information Regulations 2004

Request:

Please could you give me the number of burials and cremations from 2015 until present day. I would like this data provided as annually as opposed to a single total sum.

Response:

	Burials	Cremations
2015	508	1595
2016	452	1649
2017	454	1592
2018	450	1664
2019	403	1483
2020	414	1589

Cremations

Jan-21	Feb-21	Mar-21	Apr-21	May-21	Total
133	160	161	115	94	663

Burials

Jan-21	Feb-21	Mar-21	Apr-21	May-21	Total
39	47	46	35	35	202

Swale Borough Council

Freedom of Information Act Request

Ref: FOI No. 215

Date: 14th June 2021

Request and Response

Please supply figures for 2010 to present by year for:
A. Burials in the District
B. Cremations in the District
If you have any data for 2020/21, please supply this too by month, or total so far by year.

Note: Our response of numbers for full burials only relates to the cemeteries that are in Swale Borough Council's jurisdiction

	2010	2011	2012	2013	2014	2015
Burials	124	87	100	134	100	123
Cremations	99	84	98	87	71	80

	2016	2017	2018	2019	2020
Burials	124	87	100	134	100
Cremations	99	84	98	87	71

2021	Jan	Feb	Mar	Apr	May
Burials	124	87	100	134	100
Cremations	99	84	98	87	71

Note: We do not have a Crematorium so our response relates to the burial of cremated

Wandsworth Request for Information - 2021/4502 - Cremations & burials

I refer to your request for information received on 27/05/2021. Please see the information below in response to your request: -

Can you please provide me the total amounts of cremations and burials in the Wandsworth Borough Council jurisdiction from January 2015 through to December 2020, listed separately and annually. If it is not possible to list the cremations and burials separately, it will acceptable to list them together.

Year	Cremations	Burials	Burial of cremated remains*
2015	1483	392	133
2016	1283	347	148
2017	1232	346	142
2018	1199	317	137
2019	1154	301	141
2020	1351	367	124

Oh, and a new phenomenon appeared, 'Crisis Actors', who knew there was such a job? They were appearing in news footage in different parts of the world at the same time, same casualties in Brazil as in Italy, old footage from other news stories appearing as new, such as coffins piling up from previous disasters, why would the media need to do this? Later, we saw the same nurse appearing in pictures acting as a patient saying ' I wish to God I took the vaccines, now I'm so ill I may never see my grandchildren' -or whatever the script said.

Once you know your government, and many others around the world, are lying to you at such a monumental level, once you know they are staging a 'Casedemic', you know that anything coming next is going to be, without doubt, nefarious.

Vaccines.

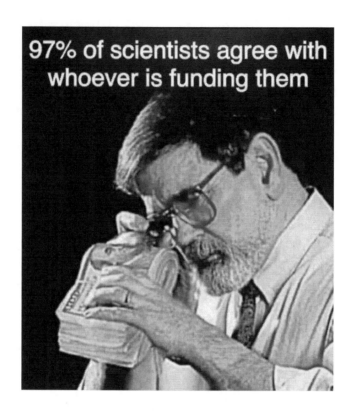

6. Why us?

Some say we were chosen, or we are 'Star Seeds', I have no idea what that is, or if we were chosen, it wasn't, therefore, my choice to become awake. It just happens, or it doesn't. I guess I allowed it to continue to happen rather than suppress it, like some people obviously have but why have hundreds of thousands of us woken up?

When I was very young, I used to get a weird sensation, it was a feeling of an immense granite-like boulder, rolling over my mind. I used to have a strange taste in my mouth, metallic, and a kind of deep, hum from a massive entity. Maybe it was as I was falling asleep; I know I always had it while alone and when quiet. I felt completely insignificant and tiny under its overwhelming power, I felt it had a presence and a meaning. It happened regularly, weekly when very young, and then more sporadic as a teenager and only twice as an adult. I never told anyone about it and thought only I was experiencing it, I felt chosen to receive it but didn't want to be. I didn't like it.

I have always felt a bit of an outsider, although I'm often very much central in small comfortable groups. For some reason, I've always felt unliked and have always fallen out with any group, like football clubs, that had its cliques, I was never in them – I can't bear sycophants.

I was a bit of a black sheep in the family and seemed to enjoy that role. I liked to antagonise – not a great trait. I would often have a hunch that something would happen, and it did. I'm prone to depression and easily latch onto something to avoid it, like alcohol.

Most people I've spoken to, on our side of the divide, seem to share these kinds of traits and histories. Most of us messed around at school, didn't try, but still came out ok with our exam results. It seems not many of us fully completed University, or the traditional post-school ones anyway. I have two medical degrees but didn't go to a conventional 'Uni'. However, we all need to have a certain ability to learn quickly, as mentioned elsewhere, we needed to be pretty clued up in Science and Geo-Politics to be able to argue our case – often getting deep into things like genetic sequencing and microbiology. Most of us seem to have had many careers and chopped around our direction in life. Most of us were probably a little left-leaning when young, before the left went mental. Most of us seemed to get into trouble a lot, we would ask 'why' a lot and irritate the receiver. We would be the ones in class to challenge the validity of something, and then find out most of the others were questioning the same but were too shy to ask. It seems that a lot of others I meet share my bad trait of saying the most inappropriate things at the wrong time, verbalising what should only be thought. I remember not long after joining the big corporate entity that ultimately made me redundant, we were called into a managers' meeting, as I sat down with the others, and the chiefs, I said, 'ooh this is a nice big room, guess it needs to be to squeeze in all the egos' – the silence had a couple of coughs in it. That was one that should have remained a thought.

Most of us can smell a rat. Is it just intuition, or do we need some proof? I needed something to confirm my intuition, just that one small thing, and then I was all in. None of us enjoy being where we are, even though we know, we are on the right side of history. Most of us are turning towards God because we have been exposed to the Devil, we know evil is in town. Some may have been 'spiritual' before, I was not and I know a lot of people who used to say they were 'spiritual' are now firmly hook, line, and sinker, caught by the devil. Jabbed. Most of us did not take one jab – we just knew. This is the thing, we knew, and we know, it's not our 'belief', or our 'view' as the normies say, patronisingly, we just KNOW!

It's an awakening we all had at some point. Once you know, you know -there is no going back.

I would bet there are thousands of people every day, having their awakening, their 'AHA experiences'. How many go the other way? How many people avoided the jabs, didn't wear masks, or joined in with the marches and protests against the globalist agendas, how many of those recently changed their minds, sought out their first Jab, and started to watch the BBC without laughing??

None, that's how many.

That proves we are right. The truth rises to the surface with zero added energy. The Truth is an energy. Lies require energy from an outside source, eventually, that source fades. We are the truth, and the truth is good. It's an easier path to travel.

Then there are other weird things like 11:11.

I always used to see this as a child, it felt very significant. Something was telling me 11:11 was important, huge, end-of-the-world stuff. It still happens and last year I glanced at my milometer in the car just as it turned 111111(0/1), I actually saw the tenths roll onto 1. I have a photo.

Some tell me it is an 'Angel Number' (?), it crops up a lot in

Telegram chats and I still fully expect something big to occur involving those numbers.

Our biggest achievement, I guess, is to override the cognitive dissonance that we have all been subjected to. We could shake it off, we fell through the net of mass formation psychosis, our intuition was stronger than the manufactured fear and subsequent need for protection.

We don't need our mummies.

We can protect ourselves thank you very much.

7. The Call-Up

The papers arrived in my head. I received the Call-up; Active Service; Time to do my Duty. It was clear and obvious. What do you do when you and your family are being attacked? Once you know, it is an immediate step into action.

This was going to be easy though, the enemy had been caught, rumbled! We can see what you're doing! The truth is out! The game is up, MoFo's!

There are thousands of people just like me, hundreds of thousands, we all got the call-up. All we have to do is notify our loved ones, our friends and colleagues and the game will be up. A simple explanation of what we have uncovered, and everyone will know. It will spread like wildfire.

Don't take the Vaccines!

Clearly, the fraudulent, PCR 'Casedemic' and media lies pushed by the governments, who were clearly controlled by darker forces, made it obvious the coming vaccines were nefarious – probably poison. Bioweapons.

Don't take the bloody Vaccines! We just had to let them know. Simple.

Something woke us up, somehow, we smelt it, and all we needed to do was wake up everyone else.

You would have thought.

I had never taken on a 'management' role in the family before but for some reason, I had been thrust into this position. I figured that I was the one 'on watch duties' as incoming was spotted, therefore, I needed to brief the team ASAP, it just happened on my watch – the others would have done the same 'obviously'. Brief them quickly, then we would all spring into action. I had played in the same football team with both my brother and my son, we always gelled, clearly cut from the same cloth, we fought together. All for one and one for all. I was filled with premature pride.

OK, so how do I inform the family? I need to calmly, but assertively, call a 'bit of a meeting' on video, WhatsApp, I believe. A 'lecture', my brother called it when confirming the time, he was always a bit funny, 'No, definitely not a lecture, but I have some really important information I need to share'.

We fixed the soonest available date and I started to collate the relevant key elements.

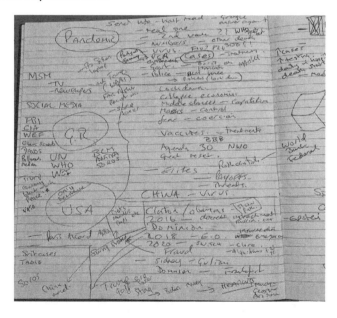

OK, Notes are ready, let's explain all to the family –
this will be easy!

Keeping it simple, what I prepared was the above.

Now, if you read this book chronologically, you would probably be thinking 'DARREN'.

Yes, I did too.

'Er, Darren, mate, I have realised you were probably right, sorry mate! I was just too wrapped up in my world to really listen to you. Thought you'd just gone mad - LOL, U always were a bit mate, I mean, Chelsea ☺ Let me know when ur next in the UK and we can catch up'

For some reason, I never got a reply. He probably changed his phone number. Oooops.

Anyway, I didn't want to copy Darren's style of delivery, too urgent, too excitable, too mental.

No, I would deliver it to my family in a calm and rational manner, keeping it light, entertaining, but effective.

The lecture – late 2020

Right, guys, I really need to explain some things to you. After two hours and two bottles of Red, I had rattled off:

lockdown, collapsing economies, middle classes, capitalism, communism, masks, control, coercion, fear, vaccines, *don't take the vaccines,* treatment, build back better, new world order, great reset, elites, Rothschilds, world bank, printing money, debt, the pope, The Vatican, payoffs, threats, cases, *don't take the vaccines*, testing, hospitals, statistics, PCR, fraud, deaths, cases, Boris, Hancock, Police, Black Lives Matter, knee taking the, protests, virus, numbers, *don't take the vaccines*, World Health Organisation, test, test, mainstream media, TV, newspapers, social media, Google, FBI, CIA, WEF, Klaus Schwab, Davos, tyranny, billionaires, Great

Reset, Agenda 21, *don't take the vaccines*, Agenda 30, Biden, laptop, Trump, wars, far-right, fascists, racists, Clinton, Obama, Dominion, Russia, impeachment, executive orders, insurrections, emergency, algorithms, fraud, Giuliani, Sidney Powell, Frankfurt, Epstein, suitcases, tabulators, Soros, China, CCP, NATO, Antifa, flu, *don't take the vaccines*, pandemic, Georgia, Arizona, Michigan, election, false flags, riots & *don't take the vaccines*.

To name a few, and in no particular order.

I thought it went well. I expected a few more questions but most were ready for bed.

Rest thy weary heads fam, Tomorrow we battle.

Don't take the vaccines. My audience for the above was only four, three did.

Enough about them, that story rolls out in the Substacks, later in the book.

Red Alert!! Incoming Vaccines from 360 Degrees. Action Stations Now.

Before embarking on a long story of what I did during these few years, I need to point out that there were thousands of us, maybe millions, all doing the same. Many were doing way much more, risking themselves and their careers. Many more than me lost so much more, such as my friend who lost her daughter. Nobody chose this nightmare, nobody really expected to be getting up to such activities, it was forced upon us, and we had to react. Again, thousands of real heroes did so much more than me and they don't seek the credit they deserve. One day they will be rewarded.

This is an account from just one small cog in a massive civilian machine grinding against the cabal – hopefully, it resonates.

Back to mid-2020

OK, how do we make sure they don't jab us? They obviously want to.

Even back then there were some heroes, a GP, a doctor, somewhere was prepared to sign exemption certificates, who knew if a certificate, a piece of paper, would do anything if they ultimately just come and kick your door down – but it was a start. Someone had the foresight, and bravery, to set up such a service. I think we found it on Parler, but maybe by then we were into some of the groups popping up on Telegram, some of them local.

It took around one second to think of our reasons why we should be medically exempt. Having a death phobia would have been good but generally, we chose allergies, asthma, and an episode of irregular heartbeats. Whatever it was, all the family had one. We were armed.

Around this time, we were reading all sorts of horror stories about the jab contents, even the PCR swab contents were reported to contain nasties. Morgellons as an example, we saw them under microscope rising up looking for victims to burrow into. Then we saw computer chips, shards of glass, horrifying hydras and other parasites, all sorts of nightmares in suspension. No idea if true at the time, but I suspect, now, that some of these stories were put out by our enemy to discredit everything negative about their jabs as theories of a conspiratorial nature. I am certain that I lost the attention from some members of the family by mentioning a few things that are now clearly wrong. You can do so much good work, put so much effort in, but one small chink of misinformation and the whole lot crumbles, and they look out for those chinks, believe me.

What I thought, partly rightly, at the time was, AstraZeneca seemed less of a genetic therapy than Pfizer, but it contained adenovirus from a Chimpanzee. Pfizer needed to be kept at minus 70 Celsius for some reason and it contained cells from a human foetus. 'There is no way any of that shit is going into me or any members of my family'. Oh, and it's still in an experimental trial period, so we would be the Guinea Pigs. Whether I was right or wrong, these vaccines were going to be nefarious as proven by the staged casedemic. I started to listen to people like Delores Cahill and Mike Yeadon to become better informed. Also, back then I listened to people like Simon Parks, Charlie Ward, and Alex Jones – fascinating, scary, implausible, plausible, I took a lot with a pinch of salt, but I certainly started to think about things very much outside of the box.

We then found out about the Vax Control Group, a fantastic idea. If Big Pharma were not going to conduct full and proper peer-reviewed, evidence-based reviews into their poisons, then we will. A 'control group' in a real-life setting was definitely required. Let's do this experiment properly. Not double-blind, of course, but it was the best we could do – and we got official-looking 'Do Not Vaccinate' ID cards.

We made new friends while rapidly losing the long-established ones. It actually became impossible to spend time with our previous friends, conversation didn't ever get very far before the wall came up, either side would activate it, but it would always appear. Also, we suddenly lost the seemingly harmless 'relaxing in front of the TV', or 'reading the paper' activities we used to enjoy – they both became intolerable, constant narratives, perpetual propaganda, unbearable.

We started to have new people around, sharing a meal, lots of wine, and amazing conversations – illegally.

At least we were not on our own. I say we, meaning myself and my wife, luckily both on the same side. We knew those who were not, and they were clearly experiencing hell.

Some friends chose the fake certificates, they cost a bomb, £400+ each, and did the job. Most of us wanted to continue to travel, us on trips to Portugal where we kept a small place, others needed to work. The drawback with this is that they were still 'playing the game' and, also, this system was integrated with the 'NHS app' – a nasty thing that wanted to trace your whereabouts and who you came into contact with – so they are now, 'officially vaccinated'. Even back then it was clear to me that one day you would need to prove you are unvaccinated – a 'pure blood' in a dystopian world. Or maybe just to prove you are safe to procreate with.

We managed to travel to Portugal a couple of times before resorting to creativity. This came when it became mandatory to produce proof of vaccine to fly. The loophole for Portugal was also proof of recovery, so at that time they accepted a natural immunity if recently recovered from 'Covid' – so you needed evidence of a PCR positive. This was before the silly lateral flow tests. We had to send the swabs off to an official lab, so virtually impossible to fake.

We had our flights booked and paid for, couldn't wait to get away from the October Grey of the UK and into the bright warm Iberian blue. It was literally a couple of weeks away. I was feeling fairly rubbish with a heavy cold when I hatched a plan. I had a hunch I would test positive, so spat on a swab and sent it off – within days, and to my delight I was Positive, Yey! I have Covid, what fun. But all four of us need 'Positives'. So, we got three more packs, I dunked one into a bit of my spit and cross-contaminated the others by rubbing them all together. We all needed to be Covid positive and officially recovered with shiny antibodies to travel. Bingo, they all came back positive! We were good to go. (Dear NHS spy, this book is fictional).

Influencers

It was just after the insurrection – the real one on November 3rd, 2020, I started to find very interesting people on YouTube or Their websites. The first that seemed to grab me was the eccentric English Simon Parkes. He had a soothing manner and made it clear he had some kind of connection with a key US intelligence operative, someone high-ranking.

Just to make it clear now, I never completely believed everything these people said, but they did make me think and they made me think about things I would never have thought of thinking about.

Back to Mr Parks, he was, sometime before, a Politician, or trying to be. I don't think he got too far because he spoke of being abducted by aliens, along with his Mother apparently. This is usually a vote loser. Anyway, he appeared in some kind of rear extension office that was fairly cluttered, and a cat would appear most times. Everything worked in terms of being an eccentric English buffoon. I was always drawn to those characters though. I, and his audience listened to his intel. He seemed connected to

Q but I don't recall him quoting Q posts – I could be wrong. We listened intently as he revealed very detailed White Hat intentions and information that confirmed their existence. We were drawing towards the sham Biden inauguration and Mr Parks was strongly hinting at a massive military operation live during the event, to mop up the whole sorry swamp. How exciting. We watched it play out – I have more details on the sham inauguration in the Q and Devolution chapters – It never happened.

The next video he put out started with Simon looking somewhat sheepish and saying, "I don't know what happened, they were going to do it, there must have been a last-minute stand down, maybe intel about a dirty bomb," 'It was going to happen, but didn't'. I was partly pissed off with him and partly compassionate as all his credibility just evaporated – although personally, I agreed that it could have easily been pulled and he could still have intel. Nevertheless, the disappointment of not watching a mind-blowing 'A-team' assault was very hard to take. I remember watching the SAS live on TV, storming the Iranian Embassy in London, I think it interrupted a major sporting event but was twenty times more exciting. Incredibly professional, no messing, flash grenades, job done – very British.

This did, though, teach me that using Q as a predictor was always going to end in disappointment, Dates and times will never be transmitted to the enemy. Q doesn't work that way, it is all about 'Future proving Past' – current actions showing in the posts, some up to 6 years back, evidence that the plan is unfurling. I think Simon's 'military' contact may well have been an Anon. Not without credibility, but perhaps not quite so direct.

One interesting point was made, though in this post-inauguration video, fellow 'conspiracy theorist' broadcaster, Charlie Ward (Dr – supposedly) had watched the whole ceremony broadcast in Spain several hours before we did. I found this suspicious as I didn't hear any other similar reports, and you would have, wouldn't you?

So, I did try Charlie, for a while. Sorry to say though, he just came across weirdly, a bit narcissistic, very religious and he had a young son who featured to show him being a family man. Something just felt off. I may be wrong. I was the same with David Icke, bless him. How hard must it be to know such massively deep and out-of-this-world facts, when nobody else does, to feel the need to wear purple and be ridiculed on TV by 'Parky'. To be honest I never really listened to him. Right now, it appears, he was very much ahead of his time and largely right with everything – bar the lizards, for now. Nothing will surprise me. He recently explained humanity's dilemma where billions are acquiescing to a few thousand wannabe dictators, either the 'poor little me' group who just do what they're told, don't make a fuss, mustn't grumble – or the ones who know they are being had, but are too feeble to fight back, all tyrannical regimes have relied on those two groups, he said. Then there are the 'awake' who do fight back, all tyrannical regimes have ultimately perished because of them.

But these people had bad PR.

This was always the trouble. When I tried to wake the Normies, there would always be something, one little thing, that renders everything I've explained in huge detail, over hours upon hours, invalid. That one little thing and suddenly they lose you, in sarcastic guffaws, walking away shaking their heads.

I had a friend – actually, the one with the matching mask and handbag set – in leopard skin. She was close to turning, I had worked on her for weeks. I got her to watch a speech by Delores Cahill the Irish Immunologist, she was brilliantly describing the anomalies with the whole Covid narrative. I knew this would fully turn her; it couldn't fail.

Then David Icke, stood next to her on the stage. 'Have you seen who she's with??', she texted, 'If she has anything to do with that fruitcake, you have lost it', 'Not interested, thanks'.

That's how quickly you lose them. Obviously to proudly don the matching leopard skin pair shows how deep she was anyway – probably unsavable.

Ironic, as Icke was a professional goalkeeper.

As we get deeper into this Clown World, the more complex the web becomes. I found myself attempting to make the headmaster of my youngest's primary school aware that he may have the 'vaccinators' coming to his school soon. What was he going to do? I asked as I preceded to inform him that it was all part of a conspiracy. He would say that he couldn't believe most countries around the world would be in on it, that they would all be acting in bad faith, that there was something planned and organised – it just doesn't happen in developed societies, he would say. I had many meetings with him and sent him a lot of info and articles and, what I considered to be undeniable proof.

The problem for any of us trying to wake the other side up, was that it was such a wide and tangled web, so many bad players and so many pieces of the jigsaw. The longer this was going on, the more difficult it was to explain. The ultimate goal when trying to red-pill someone is to maintain your credibility, your trustworthiness, and your sanity. You have to capture their attention with some undeniable facts and then fill in the blanks to further cement belief – in you, and the story. You have to provide the dots that they may know to be real, or accept likely, and help them join those dots.

What happens in general is that you get about 30 seconds in, and they already have you down as one of those 'anti-vaxers' they've read about, or been warned about. In fact, you are often lucky to get that 30 seconds in.

I will talk about organised protests and marches later, and that there were, and still are, a lot of organised 'outreach' activities to try and offer the public information that may just prime their alarm clock. One such event took place outside a technical college that my daughter attended, I would usually be present with this group (maybe 15 people), but for obvious reasons thought better of it on this occasion. The noble aim was to inform the teenagers about the risks of the 'Vaccines' and the fact they were not going to be fully informed, so they wouldn't be able to give 'informed consent' – basic stuff, coming from a good place, purely for their safety.

My daughter came home a little later than usual showing me a text she received from her college.

It went something like this; 'You may be aware of a group of Anti-Vaxers outside our college today. Do not engage, do not speak to them, it will play into their hands'.

IT WILL PLAY INTO THEIR HANDS!!! Unbelievable! I found this statement mind-blowing, what exactly is their mindset here? How evil do they think 'Anti-Vaxers' are for fuck's sake? This really let me know how deeply they had been brainwashed, how entrenched they had become.

So, the students left their classrooms at the end of the day, eager to see these crazy predators, they were fully charged and full of excitable hormones, ready to fight, to scream and shout and vent all that pent-up irrational teen energy. So, they did, they surrounded the good-intentioned folk and spat at them (literally spat) with the 'most vile' abuse imaginable – all stoked up by the teachers. This is how it works.

This was my email to them

Hello - please can you ensure this email gets to the appropriate person.

RE Anti-Vaxer's Friday 4th

I am a parent of a student who is doing very well and is very happy at YOUR COLLEGE.

In fact, I would say he is now blossoming after suffering severe depression last year.

Unfortunately, an incident has created great anxiety and a very low mood.

Please read all of this as there is a question at the end that I would like an answer to.

I am remaining anonymous to keep his privacy.

On Friday he was sent a text advising him NOT to engage with the so-called 'Anti-Vaxers'.

You actually said 'do not play into their hands' – what do you mean here??

The text implied that there was something very negative about the 'Anti-Vaxers' and they should not take any information from them.

You must know that it may well prove to be a 'life or death' decision for a teenager to take these injections.

They are at virtually zero risk from Covid. No healthy child has died from Covid 19 in the UK.

Most 'anti-vaxers' are pro-vaccines, but pro the ones that work and are fully tested for safety.

These injections are NOT normal vaccines, they are still experimental until 2023 and are, in fact, a gene therapy that does not prevent infection or transmission but permanently alters a previously healthy immune system. Some 1700 people in the UK have died shortly after taking them as reported by the yellow card system (known to be only reporting 1-10% of all adverse reactions). There is a spike in childhood deaths since the rollout, over 50% above the 5-year average, hospitals are becoming full of the vaccinated with a large increase of unusual blood clotting disorders and myocarditis. Research this before dismissing it.

How about also researching if the PCR test produces 90%+ false positives, and therefore incorrect numbers of 'cases'- where did the flu go? Why no more burials and cremations in 2020 than average? Etc. I mean, you are a college, you should be able to research independently, right?

These children need to make an INFORMED decision to give INFORMED consent.

The people that you call 'Anti-Vaxers' are purely trying to help the children – without the 'harassment' as reported- by giving them an opportunity to obtain balanced information. They are mainly educated and professional people. I challenge you to find one piece of information they give that has been peer-reviewed as scientifically incorrect.

The government and the media suppress and censor anything that may put children off taking the injections for reasons you should question – the JVCI told the government not to push it onto the children as there were enough concerns about the risks. Yet they are pushing hard. Why? (You may ask).

I am aware that some teachers make it very clear they object to Anti-Vaxers, (and presumably the unvaccinated?), this leads to coercion by students' peers and that is highly unfair on the children who have decided not to take the risk. There is a narrative that encourages hate against innocent people who choose not to take the jab. I urge you to ensure YOUR COLLEGE does not participate in this blatant discrimination. My child received aggressive words from his student friends when they found he was unvaccinated, this has caused a high level of anxiety and depression. This is your fault by setting the narrative with that text, it primed the students to be highly charged.

The person who sent the text and the teachers who impose their narrow and ill-informed view may well find themselves guilty, in the future, of a crime by spreading misinformation that endangers lives.

The people who you call anti-vaxers are purely trying to save lives- they do not enjoy standing in the cold and rain taking abuse. I suggest you take a different approach to them quickly.

How are you going to prevent further abuse and discrimination against my child? I welcome an urgent response.

Please confirm receipt of this email

Thank you.

Parent

This was their response (which I found very honest and well thought out, so I thanked them in reply), glad to see they were probably wondering who my 'Son' was):

Thank you for your email and apologies we have not until now replied – we have had a very demanding week. We acknowledge the concerns you raise about college messaging to its students. We'll take your points on board when we make our communications decisions. When we arrived having been informed of the demonstration along the length of one side of the college and 10 minutes before all our students finished their lessons for the day and week, we saw a heated debate between a protestor and a police officer with raised voices and some physical engagement and didn't know what to make of it and felt we needed to get a communication out quickly to our students to avoid any escalations.

Perhaps our experiences in the past with Abort66 protesting on a very regular basis outside the college about a topic which distressed many of our students (along with the images they used), causing some triggers by students of aggravation and disorder have led us to be over-cautious. The demonstration last Friday was actually very well conducted on all sides and there were no frictions or problems arising at all between our community and demonstration, for which OUR COLLEGE is grateful.

If you could pass this information to your son for reassurance, we'd be grateful. If your son has any support needs which we are able to help with as his education provider and he isn't accessing these already, I'd encourage him to seek that support. We do not and hold anything against any of our students or treat them with bias because of their views around this matter. Indeed, we don't need to know unless it is a barrier to understanding and providing support and any complaint made is treated confidentially and not shared with other staff unless the complaint is relevant to them. You do not need to send your complaint to us anonymously because of this.

I hope your son can recover and get better and I hope we are able to help if we can.

Many thanks,

THE COLLEGE

I hope, in this case, that some minds were changed when they took the time and trouble to formulate their reply.

Your target is often ready primed, if not by teachers, but by the mainstream media. We know their game.

So, back to the point. If you have got through that initial 30 seconds, it often gets worse. This is it, you are live, don't mess up, don't hesitate, don't say 'um', You got one shot and you are working against the body language that is hitting you hard. The body language that tells you they think you are a nutter, a fruitcake, gullible, one of those tin foil hat wearers. Just a little eyebrow twitch is enough. As you work your way through your pitch, you feel a bead of sweat, you lose your script, you go blank with the numbers – it's Dragon's Den / The Sharks Tank – they are looking at you, thinking, 'he's mad', you start thinking 'he thinks I'm mad' – and you end up sounding like you are mad.

This is the level we have to operate at, Dragon's Den, yet none of us chose to be on this side of the studio, standing and delivering, whilst inside withering and wilting. It's really bloody hard. Most of us fail and none of us were trained – this is an information war; we have to get it right.

I started to listen to presenters from the US, it was becoming clear to me that the only thing preventing total global tyranny was the 2nd amendment and threatening that was the radical left's election steal. The US was the last bastion of defence, if the US falls, the world falls.

I was very impressed with Steve Bannon, even though I felt his work with Cambridge Analytica was equally dishonest regarding election fraud – but then realised you needed to fight fraud with fraud, clearly social media was being manipulated to influence voters, at this point I had no idea quite how controlled it was, going right to the heart of Government and three letter agencies. I would also listen to Mike Adams, the Health Ranger. He was very direct in presenting the clear and present danger we were in. he provided a lot of useful information for me to use as ammo when playing my part in this information war. Real science. However, he also became quite negative to the point where I was becoming depressed and losing hope.

If you are fighting a war, you need hope. You need to see a light at the end of a tunnel if you are to maintain momentum. You also need to give some hope to your fellow warriors. Yes, we used such terms as the battle intensified, it was getting nasty, people hated us.

Really hated us.

They hated us because the good people they knew on the television, the people they grew up with, and respected, were saying this about us;

- *"You're willing to walk amongst us, Unvaccinated, you are the enemy" Simmons (Kiss my ass)*
- *"When are we gonna stop putting up with idiots in this country and say it's mandatory to get vaccinated? Fuck them, Fuck their freedom." Stern (he said Sternly)*
- *"Love the idea of COVID vaccine passports for everywhere: Flights, clubs, gyms, shops. It's time COVID denying, Anti-Vaxer loonies had their bull-shit bluff called." Morgan (OK Mr Potato Head)*
- *"Don't have the vaccine, can't go to supermarket... Can't go to the ball game... can't go to work... No shirt, No shoes, No service!" Lemon (Lemonaids anyone?)*
- *"Who gets on [Sic] ICU bed? Vaccinated person, come right in. Unvaccinated person who gobbled horse goo... Rest in peace, Wheezy." Kimble (It's AN ICU bed, not ON -you've got one job....)*
- *"Screw your freedom!" Schwarzenegger (Gonad the Barbarian)*

- *"In all my time in public life. I have never come across a group so blinkered and dangerous as Anti-Vaxers."* Hancock (the voice of [T]reason)
- *"It's time to send unvaccinated citizens to Jail."* Penn (100 million new prisoners? It's a Plan Stan!)
- *"The best gift we can offer our families this Christmas is to refuse to meet them."* Ransen (That's Death! – you need to be a UK viewer of a certain age)
- *"To love one another, as Jesus said, get vaccinated, get boosted."* Welby (It was a lesser-known Jesus quote)
- *"You have no right not to take a Covid vaccine, you have no right not to wear a mask, you have no right to open up your business"* Dershowitz (It's in Blacks Dictionary somewhere)
- *"I don't want the unvaccinated sitting next to me in a theatre, near me, or on the same train carriage."* Curry (the feeling's mutual, Shedder)
- *"All the unvaccinated are idiots!"* Blair (Sir! Sir, He called me an idiot!)
- *"We are going to end this pandemic by proceeding with the vaccination... There is still a part of the population fiercely against it. They don't believe in science or progress and are very often misogynistic and racist... They take up some space. This leads us, as a leader and as a country, to make a choice. Do we tolerate these people?* Trudeau (he sang, with Minstrel hands, cute little face all 'blacked up')
- *"The vaccine's been tested for all ethnicities, it's safe"*
  "Trust the experts, don't trust your mate down the pub or conspiracies online" Henry (it's the way you tell 'em – the

comedians' comedian't)

- "I hope all out there in the Twitterverse that at the moment of your death, your final words are not I wish I had gotten the vaccine." Curtis (does she really hope this, though? Me saying the word 'gotten' on my deathbed is very remote)
- "It's time to punish Britain's five million vaccine refuseniks" "Why shouldn't we curb some of their freedoms?" Neil (Damn, I was just fantasizing over you whipping me with a Cat o'Nine Tails)
- "It's only the idiots who don't take the vaccine, the moronic idiots" Whale (Beached Whale)

...and then there was the grotesque James Corden and Ariana Grande, 'singing in the rain' style video of their song 'No Lockdowns Anymore' – I was literally blindsided – was this really real? So bizarre that I am surprised to confirm it wasn't just a disturbing dream. Can I quote the line *'shout out to our favourite MD, Anthoneeee Faucheeeee'* without vomiting? Nope.

And what were the Governments telling their people? On TV, Radio, Billboards, Busses...

- We're all in it together.
- Look him in the eyes and tell him you always keep safe distance.
- Look her in the eyes and tell her you never bend the rules.
- Look him in the eyes and tell him the risk isn't real.
- COVID-19 vaccine - The NHS will get in touch when it's your turn to be vaccinated.

- Act like you've got it. Anyone can spread it.
- We're doing our part. Are you doing yours?
- Stay home. Will you bring the virus into your community?
- Local COVID Alert Level - High
- You must only meet people socially in groups of up to six.
- 1 in 3 people are asymptomatic.
- Follow social distancing when you meet, work from home.
- Stay alert. Control a virus, Save lives.
- Stay in your bubble.
- Wash your hands maintain physical distance.
- Protect the elders. Keep safe.
- Help our heroes. Protect the NHS.
- If you go out, you can spread it, people will die.
- Anyone can get it. Anyone can spread it.
- Stay inside. For you, for them. For us.
- Victory begins at home.
- Back to normal is up to you.
- Self-isolate and get tested if you have symptoms.
- You are the frontline.
- To the doctors, thank you for leaving your homes to keep us safe in ours.
- The vaccines are safe, effective, and used worldwide.
- They keep you, your family, and your community safe.
- Get boosted now.
- Every adult in the country now needs to get a COVID-19 booster vaccine because two doses do not give you enough protection against catching Omicron.
- Your loved ones need you. Get the COVID-19 vaccine to make

sure you can be there for them.

- You need two doses for maximum protection. We'll let you know when your next vaccine is ready for you.
- Thank you, NHS, I'll get my COVID vaccine.
- Boost your power. Get vaccinated so we can all get back to normal.
- Wear a mask after you're vaccinated, they protect against any strain of the coronavirus in spite of genetic mutations.
- Be a vaccine hero.
- Roses are red, COVID-19 cases levels are too, vaccines will make you immune, after shot number 2... yes, this was real.

I could go on. An awful lot of 'you's' in there, subliminal guilt bombs? They did think they were clever, didn't they?

In 2012, Obama passed a bill that made it legal to propagandise its citizens. They could say whatever they wanted; it didn't need to be true.

None of this needed to be true, they could always say it was for the greater good. It was as true as TV adverts are, like 'killing up to 99% of germs', the key bit is 'up to', could be 46, or 63%, who knows, it just won't be over 99. Or 8 out of 10 say they prefer SuperGum, but don't say what the alternative is, maybe the question was; Do you prefer SuperGum or Herpes? You may get 2 weirdos.

So, the government telling us we needed to be vaccinated to save someone else who is also vaccinated is as true as telling you to wear a nappy to stop someone else shitting themselves.

Nevertheless, it worked and therefore we who refused the vaccines and masks were hated by those who complied.

This is what we were, and still are, up against.

The Health Ranger led me to Alex Jones, but I just couldn't get past his voice. I'm easily put off. Like my adversaries across the divide, it doesn't take much for me to shut down. As bad as it sounds, I have little tolerance, little scope for attention when there is a distraction. I found the same with RFK Jr but forced myself to overcome the obvious vocal issues as he must have done himself – to his immense credit.

Then came Scott McKay, The Patriot Streetfighter. I really loved his patriotic intro, very anthemic, and very military, quoting words from the Constitution. I have a lot of admiration for him and his shows. Mainly for his stressing to 'Hold the Forking Line', to stop 'the people' from taking up arms and creating the civil war that the Cabal clearly wanted. He would quote Q repeating his mantra – everyone needed to stay calm, and just fight back with words and information. Clearly, McKay loved his guns, and pictures of him suggested a military background, but he could just be a regular redneck, I wasn't sure, but didn't care. His shows made me feel bigger and more confident. I cooled on him a bit when he started touring and had his own tour bus that looked like it was previously owned by Evel Knievel. Nothing wrong with that though.

Then I found Dave.

Big dramatic Bam, Bam, Bam, Dum Dum Dum, Dum intro with the uplifting transposition before the ever consistent *"Hiiiiii (low to high) and Welcome, you're listening to the X22 report, my name's Dave and this episode three thousand two hundred and two Bee-aaand today's date is November second twenty twenty-three and the title of this episode is... ....*

Then comes the advert about Belly Fat or the Fighter-Fire-Flash-

Light, or annoying wrinkles.

Stick with it, that's what I learned because a gem of a show follows.

"Let's into the economic collapse, political and geopolitical news – Now the deep state, the corrupt politicians, Big Tech, the fake news, the puppets masters, they are now panicking... ..."

Dave is my hero and saviour, he kept me sane for three years and counting. He gives me hope and always ends his show saying *"The Patriots are in control"* – sometimes it doesn't feel like it but, ultimately that is exactly what I believe – see my chapters on Q and Devolution. We all need reassurance from time to time, we all need to keep our peckers up and we need to support each other, this is a war of attrition. Dave deserves a medal, honestly, a real one, in fact, he deserves much more, I rarely hear him down or in despair. He must be drained and burnt out at times, but I have not known him to take a break, maybe the odd day, but not a well-deserved holiday to my knowledge. This man is the equivalent of the BBC's Home Service for the troops – before the BBC became the enemy.

Somehow, he has prepared for, written, and recorded two different shows, the A (Financial) and the B (geopolitical), five times per week since 2008, and he also does a regular interview show, in total I estimate he has done well over six thousand shows.

Don't touch that dial

I found myself calling TV and radio shows, just couldn't bear their utter nonsense. You still hear it now, the news readers telling you something you know to be complete propaganda, utter horseshit, brainwashing narratives, you know this, and yet, unbelievably, people believe it. It makes you scream at the TV, or the radio in the car. I wonder how many times I've been seen shouting at my dashboard whilst waiting at the traffic lights.

The first one was with GB News, Dan Wooton was presenting, he had a series of dire warnings coming from the government and terrified people calling in. Everyone was preparing for the next bubonic plague, the black death, the Spanish Flu, we were all going to die. I suffer from social anxiety, the thought of public speaking terrifies me, I have panic attacks, go bright red, sweat like a pig, and forget everything I'm one second away from saying. However, I really did not see anyone around me being sick. This was very early in 2020, was having serious doubts but was yet to have my big awakening supermarket experience, which must have been days away. Nevertheless, I was so flabbergasted by the hysteria, I found myself waiting on the line, Dan was coming to me next. Gulp, I'm about to go on TV.

Dan was really nice, it was very brief, I just said I don't think this Covid thing will amount to much and everything will be normal pretty soon. I got the sense that he rather agreed. A few days later the UK went pandemic crazy. My big, televised' pronouncement was wrong, how many people cast their mind back to that dickhead on TV telling us nothing was coming – we had a weatherman famously telling the country to not worry, a hurricane is not coming – a few days before the country was flattened. I think it killed his career, mine never started, but for a short while, I felt his pain.

On November 4th, 2020, I called into a radio show, wild with rage. I was shaking with vitriol listening to a stream of over-excited

Trump haters, jubilant at the success of Joseph R Biden. The racist, orange-faced crook had been defeated, the people have spoken, the people are free from his right-wing rhetoric, the future is Gay (in the old sense). I believe it was LBC and the presenter was such a narcissistic legend, like a Brazilian footballer, he only needed one name – Christo. Christo, what a twat he was.

'What makes you think it was stolen then? How would you know? How do you know more than us, and the good people who run the elections? This is the USA, not some tin pot banana republic, these elections were the most secure in history.' He went on and on, when I started to speak, he cut into me, let's hear what Nigel thinks in Nottingham shall we?', 'Nigel what do you think about this callers' views?' Nigel would agree with Christo, and they took it in turns to say 'nonsense', 'rubbish' 'are you far right, you are, aren't you, well, you have no place in modern Britain' etc. What was interesting though was my wife was listening to the radio in the room next door, she could hear me and the radio. I was invited to explain my views and as I was talking, I was being faded out so our friend Nigel could speak. On radio, I didn't complete one sentence, yet in my office I was doing very well, putting great arguments and facts across. Christo was a bully, patronising and disingenuous, he questioned my mental health when I told him I was being silenced whenever I gave details of the evidence (I already had a lot only 12 hours after the event), he told me I hadn't mentioned anything of any substance. Clearly, their script had already been written, he was using terms such as 'baseless' and 'unfounded' – we heard that a lot in the coming months.

Before I knew it, I was off air and Christo was playing 'Celebration' by Kool and the Gang. Yahoo.

Jan 6ᵗʰ

After the disbelief of the election night/week the previous
November, we were anticipating some major shenanigans on
January the sixth, the day that the results of the election were to
be accepted by Capitol Hill. A lot of us knew that Mike Pence could
decide to send the Electoral College votes back to the legislators,
and we were expecting him to do so due to the overwhelming
evidence of fraud and irregularities. This has since been disputed,
but most commentators at the time appeared to act like they
thought it possible, and the fact that one year later Democrat
senators tried to reform the act to ensure a vice president couldn't
interrupt the process, indicates that, previously, he could. Typical
nonsense. Trump was also hinting this was an expectation but not
publicly calling for it. I started to have my doubts and we were
speculating if he was working for the Deep State.

I was very much in two minds sometime later, having watched
Christopher Miller, the acting US Secretary of Defence, thank Mike
Pence for his leadership during one of the most intense military
operations over 'the last few months' – those of us following the
Devolution series viewed that as very much evidence of a White
Hat operation. We shall see.

I can be swayed by some very benign things, such as a fly landing
on his head, and staying there, during a vice presidential debate –
it was almost trying to tell us something. Maybe it just didn't like
the smell of Kamala Harris.

Pence chose not to interrupt the process; he allowed the Electoral College Votes and received 'some kind of' secret coin for doing so – a medal for courage. There were objections raised by various senators and often the Senate would retire to consider, but it always looked in vain. The controlled players were doing as told. The corrupt Dems and the RINO's, bullies but cowards, the Lion without a roar, without courage.

I'm not going to go on too much about the 'storming of the Capitol' other than, initially, I did think it was 'the people' snapping and fighting back against a corrupt bunch of liars and thieves. If I could watch it happen blatantly in the UK, then surely enough in the US would have also, and would have been so incensed as to barge their way in and physically remove the invaders – the real insurrectionists. I would not have blamed them.

But Trump was telling them to go home in peace. I felt sorry for him giving his final speech before they officially declared him done. It was behind very thick glass, he arrived late, in my opinion, to stop people from gathering at the doors of Capitol Hill. Of course, he was not inciting a violent insurgency. He posted clear instructions on Twitter, but we now find out – thanks to the Twitter Files - those posts were suppressed intentionally.

We saw it on TV, it looked like swathes of red-hatted MAGA supporters were breaking their way in, mayhem, I became rather excited, calling my friends and brother – 'Watch the news, the people are taking back their country, this is monumental!'

Then I saw Antifa - we saw them before, creating all the riots to discredit Trump's presidency – controlled opposition, paid actors - changing from their black clothes, putting on MAGA hats, and lifting Trump flags before running towards the doors, I saw Police seemingly invite people in, I saw good people shouting at the armed Police to 'take action', to protect the building – they didn't and wouldn't. I knew Nancy declined the offer of thousands of National Guard and I could see this was yet another staged event.

It seemed the last hope came and went when the GOP (Republican) leader, Mitch McConnell – old turtle-neck - stood to make his statement condemning efforts to overturn the results. He did this after the 'so-called' storming of the Capitol and immediately called it an insurrection by Trump supporters, like his script was already written.

Importantly, before he spoke, he nervously looked behind at someone sat looking back at him, this person appeared to be making hand gestures 'of the Illuminati kind', in a threatening manner, it happened several times, McConnel was visibly shaken when seeing them – he looked haunted. For me, this was a significant moment, it made me shiver like seeing a ghost – terrifying and, unfortunately, conclusive proof of systematic evil – the men in black. Just my interpretation but nobody will convince me it was a nothing burger. This was undeniable proof that we were up against a very dark force.

I instantly set up a Jan 6th evidence telegram channel, knowing that at some point in history, we will need every piece of evidence to prove this was an inside job. In my haste, I set it up with the wrong date – Jan 6th, 2020, should have been 2021, only realising last year when I was surprised to see only a handful of contributions.

Luckily, The US Military, NSA, and Space Force had a backup system in place, just in case mine failed.

Poster Boy

I couldn't do nothing. I couldn't – even though I was still technically on Furlough with my 'well up' corporate position – I had to do something. People had to be told. Surely, they would wake up once they see what I know, when they know what I see. I found a great resource, 'StopWorldControl.Com' a website with the tools I needed – ready-made templates for flyers with QR codes. Succinct information, simple and direct with all the backup data instantly downloadable. Brilliant. I chose two or three and had several printed. I was also aware of a good one from WorldDoctorsAlliance.Com, also with QR codes to good information – perfect. I made up some flour and water paste and embarked on a few weeks of splattering them around a mile radius of my home, at night with my hood up.

The first night was blustery, by the sea, loads of people by day, perfect. I noticed a few cameras up high on poles so worked out the best locations. Walking up and down with posters up my jacket and a tub of homemade glue. Not easy, I realised that I needed three hands, one to hold the poster, one to hold the brush, and one to hold the pot. There were other ways that involved a foot and the floor, but my knees were killing me, and I just looked too odd, bending down every 3 minutes, you can only pretend to tie your shoelaces once or twice. So, I worked a hybrid where I placed the pot between my knees, leaned against the lamp post (which was the allocated poster spot) in a pseudo-casual way, painted the lamppost with glue, and splatted the printed paper on top, gathering myself up quickly and moving on to the next. My fingers were covered in glue and all I could do was lick them clean – a bit of flavouring next time, I thought.

The next day I thought I would go for a bit of a jog, to inspect my work and see the crowds gathered around each lamppost. No crowds. It had rained. All bar three posters had slipped down the poles and were sodden, 50% bubbling glue, and 50% rainwater. The three that remained were intact. I stopped and watched for a while; people just walked straight past. Nobody was interested. I watched for about ten minutes then he stopped, a chap with a beard and a yellow jacket, not only did he read it, but he got his phone out and pointed it at the QR code. Success-ish.

I thought it had a one-in-twenty success rate. Then I realised that one person could possibly read all the information on the website, have his 'awakening' moment, and eventually wake 19 other people, meaning a kind of 100% success.

The next day, those three posters had been picked off and ripped down, the glue looked resilient, they obviously had a hard time, little bits of QR or Text remained but clearly, someone didn't like them. Bastards.

Next time, I used a glue stick. Easier to use when applied to the surface rather than the paper poster, you just crumple the paper, it doesn't look professional. I was a professional.

Suddenly, I was an undercover vigilante commando, working at night, it was exciting and addictive, I couldn't stop popping out even if it were to get a couple up. I would also go out at dusk, just couldn't wait until full darkness, sometimes people saw, I didn't care but made very long and strange detours on my way home. I was surely being followed and tracked.

Every time I stuck them up, the next day someone pulled them down.

Obviously, the council had created a job – 'flyer un-sticker-upper'. Or 'flyer sticker downer'? Not sure of the official title, but we had established a push-me-pull-me relationship. Tom and Jerry.

Then they released the vaccines and started to push them into the schools for over 12s.

Now things were becoming urgent. The schools will be encouraging their pupils to take them, the government already declared the decision would rest with the pupils, parents could not override them. I knew they would not be able to make an informed decision, because they won't be informed.

I had to make some posters and get them up in the streets around the schools, making sure the kids saw them on their way in.

This time, I wasn't going to mess around with homemade glue or even the glue sticks, it had to be a swift operation. Sticky-backed A5 flyers were the answer, I found a printer who didn't care what he printed, as long as you paid cash – fine by me, and he could do peel-off sticker versions. Brilliant.

I wrote the key message and placed an order of 200, that would cover the 2 secondary schools nearest to me. We are talking September 2001. I had already been involved in activities against the vaccine rollout for adults which is a whole new chapter.

The stickers were done, I collected them and was pleased with how they looked. A bold red border made them stand out, and there was a QR 'read me' box that led to a dedicated website with information and facts for teenagers.

The flyer read:

COVID VAX FACTS. (12 yrs +)

1. **It will not stop you catching the virus.**
2. **It will not stop you passing it on (so it doesn't work).**
3. **You have a 99.9996% chance of surviving COVID.**
4. **Almost 2000 UK people have died after the injections so far.**
5. **It permanently weakens your immune system.**
6. **It is still experimental until 2023. Nobody knows the long-term effects.**
   What reason would you have to take it?

I set my alarm for 2 AM. I was going into a very built-up suburban area and needed to get as many done as humanly possible before dawn, and before my daughters woke to find out what I was up to. Neither of them went to those schools due to their age, that wasn't the point. They were very concerned about their dad, who not long ago was high up in the corporate world and was now behaving like Swampy – a scruffy UK eco-warrior, obsessed with conspiracy theories, falling out with their friends' dads, and acting oddly.

It's very light, I thought as I parked up, the streetlights seemed to be everywhere, everything was orange but certainly not dark enough not to be seen. The mission had started, no turning back. I placed a wad of flyers into a bag and got out, making my way up to the first school. I would target all the main approach roads from around half a mile radius. The first car to pass me was the Police, they looked at me as they passed, I tried to look like I was on my way home from a night out clubbing (as if!) They continued and all was quiet. I was right next to a big green 'telecom company' cable box, perfect.

Pulling out the first flyer, whilst scanning for cars and people, I started to pick at the corner of the backing. I still bite my fingernails, obviously of a nervous disposition, and this was a perfect reminder of the drawbacks, it took ages to prise up enough to get a holding. OK, gotcha, now whip off the back and stick it up quickly. I whipped it off, but it felt all wrong, too 'light', too easy, too quick.

Looking down, to my horror I saw in my hand a strip of backing paper full width but only a couple of centimetres in height. For no possible reason, the backing had been scored into six individual sections – why? Why would you do that? Who thought that a good idea? Has there ever been anyone in the history of the sticker-making profession who had a clamour of disgruntled customers complaining of single-sheet sticker backings?

Bollocks! This meant for every flyer, I had to try and pick at a corner 'forever', six times before affixing it. I can't begin to really explain how difficult this was, it was windy, sometimes it was too dark to see, the bits I had removed were now sticky, they were now flappy sections that would either stick to my hand or another part of itself.

I was so cross with the printer that I started not to care if any early morning dog walker saw me, and several did. I think, in two hours, I probably managed to put up 60 flyers. My pockets were rammed full of strips of backing and failed flyers stuck fast (to themselves). I got back to the car and had a little drive around to inspect my work – actually, it was pretty good, they were noticeable and frequent. I had a couple of hours to sleep before the school run. The kids would never know my secret nightlife.

Dropping my kids off allowed me to drive past opportunities to assess my work. I saw some kids stopping and reading, then mostly laughing with each other, didn't know what to make of that but at least they drew some attention. Then at the bottom of one road near a junction, I saw a teacher (I presume) trying to scrape one off the lamppost that was its' very temporary host. He was using his keys and having great difficulty being the hero he thought he was. I beeped at him as I passed, my beep meant 'you c*nt', he waved back 'thank you, yes, I'm the man'. That evening on school pickup I noticed half of them had been scraped off, but they left a lot of the flyer intact, proving the quality of the glue. After a week there were loads of remnants of posters surrounding the two schools. In a way, I felt they had more impact – they showed some people really didn't want you to read the message.

I heard there was a date announced for the school jab rollout, I became overwhelmed with the reality that they were doing this to the children – and purposely cutting parents out of the decision – God knows what propaganda was happening in the classrooms to coerce.

Of course, I was not alone, thousands, if not, hundreds of thousands of people up and down the country were taking action, either as individuals, or in groups. Telegram was awash with planned action and the material to help do the job. I found a very good handout that I thought should be given to the kids directly and for them to be advised to pass on to their parents. It was a form, to be read and completed for both the recipient of the vaccine and the 'vaccinator' clinician. On the back there were QR codes for lots of CDC, Government, and NHS sites that actually contained some of the more worrying statistics – it was all credible information, well, credible enough for those who trust their people in power.

The title was '**INFORMED CONSENT** FOR COVID-19 VACCINATION'. The point was to focus the attention of both participants to ensure the right information was provided so informed consent can be given. A series of statements were followed by tick boxes for each statement, and both would tick to confirm they understood.

It was to provide protection for both parties, but also to try and wake up the vaccinators.

The statements were:

- **Unlike traditional vaccines, the vaccines being used for COVID-19 ("the COVID-19 vaccines") instruct the body's cells to create the SARS-CoV-2 spike protein.**
- **The COVID-19 vaccines may reduce severity of symptoms if the patient gets COVID-19, but may not prevent them from getting COVID-19 nor from passing it on.**
- **Although alternative treatments are available, the COVID-19 vaccines have been granted. Emergency Use Authorization, so require less comprehensive clinical data.**

- By 18th August 2021, of the 47,460,526 People that had received at least one jab, there had been 1609 deaths (0.0003%) 351,404 adverse reports (0.7%), and 1,165,636 adverse reactions (2.5%) officially reported. Actual figures may be 10 times higher. Adverse reactions were reported more often in younger people than in older adults.
- Adverse reactions to the COVID-19 vaccines include, but are not limited to, strokes, blindness, deafness, clotting, miscarriages, anaphylaxis and cardiovascular disorders.
- We will not know what the possible long-term effects of the COVID-19 vaccines may be (EG infertility) until after the studies of the clinical trials conclude in 2023.
- The manufacturers of the COVID-19 vaccines are immune from civil liability.
- As of the 11th of January 2021, the average age of death in the UK with COVID-19 was 83.
- From the 29th of June 2020 to the 12th of May 2021, in the UK, the chance of dying *with* COVID-19 (the crude mortality rate) may be less than that of dying from the COVID vaccines.
  - Under-fives: around 0.0002%
  - 5-9 years-old: around 0.0001%
  - 10-19 years-old: around 0.0006%
  - 20-29 years-old: around 0.002%
  - 30-39 years-old: around 0.008%
  - 40-49 years-old: around 0.02%
  - 50-59 years-old: around 0.07%
  - 60-69 years-old: around 0.2%

- o **70-79 years old: around 0.5%**
- o **80 years-old and above: around 2.3%**
- **The patient/carer does not feel coerced to accept an experimental COVID-19 vaccine, and understands they are free to postpone or decline treatment at any time.**

Both were then invited to sign that they agreed to move forward with 'informed consent'.

I spent a couple of days handing them out to students, suggesting they give them to their parents. A lot of them seemed grateful. But I was also ignored by many, and I was also approached by a teacher to ask me what I was doing and what I was handing out. At that point, I thought it best to make myself disappear fairly quickly. I didn't show him what I was handing out, probably he saw some that had been given to students. Who knows? The students were obviously being warned about such dangerous literature being handed out, some were obviously reporting back. Also, the last thing I wanted was to be a suspicious loiterer outside schools.

I decided to place the remaining forms in a cardboard box placed on a bench, where a lot of the kids congregated. All I could do was make them available.

Ten minutes before school was out, I left the box and sat in my car at a distance to watch. The vast majority just walked straight past, maybe one in five would stop, stoop, and walk on, maybe one in ten would pick one up, half of those would be seen to chuck them away 30 seconds later. Then one 'teacher's pet', goody bloody two-shoes, and a rather fat girl, picked up the entire box, about turned, and 'off footed it' back to school. How much more 'pleased with herself' could she look? Obviously now a prefect, or milk monitor, something prestigious.

8. The People Rise Up

The great unforeseen for all of us three years ago was that we were suddenly going to become specialists in the worlds of Immunology, Virology, Micro-Biology, Geo-Politics, History, Chemistry, Marxism, Meteorology, Physics, Psychology, and the Art of Warfare – to name a few. We needed to know our stuff as we were about to come face to face with experts, and know-alls who were also angry, nasty, and scared - as I said before they hated us. We must be prepared.

24th April 2021. London.

A last-minute decision found me on a train to London, they threatened train strikes for that day, knowing full well a lot of people were planning on descending on the capital – it was the Unite for Freedom event, a lot of trains were indeed cancelled but people found a way to get there. The train was packed, and it was noticeable instantly that we were all going to the same event and all awake to the cabal. What I noticed for the first time, though, was we were all in an echo chamber, all stating the same facts to each other and offering a lot of 'did you knows'. However, it was equally important for us to know the size of our army and to pick up new names to look out for on Rumble or Telegram. By the time we drew into London, I decided to disembark one stop early to take a walk and clear my head – it was intense, already - and that was with my own team!

Getting nearer Parliament Square I could hear a throb of drums and people, it was a beautiful sunny day. I noticed caravans of police vans, lined up in side streets all full of silly-looking plod, they must have been scared. I saw centurions of them with shields and batons practicing a coordinated brisk walk to nowhere – they were ready. The atmosphere was charged with pre-battle tension, but our side were all smiles. It was a happy, wonderful event.

Parliament Square was rammed, I found myself standing on the feet of a ten-foot-tall Mahatma Gandhi, behind a speaker's stage with a view 'to live for' – thousands of flags, smoke, signs, colours, just people, all ages, all types, but people who won't take the crap anymore. I met Kate Shemirani and Delores Cahill, two very vocal and brave speakers who I would meet again in different arenas.

This was also the first time I heard and met Remeece, a Jamaican guy who produced his tune 'DONT TEK DI VACCINE' and played it loudly on a massive speaker on wheels. It gave a powerful vibe and energy to these events, a kind of strength, like the 'extra man' the Kop give Liverpool football club.

He would turn up at all marches, and protests and often just turn up outside the schools with his own outreach operation, his freedom movement, the kids loved him, he had a great smile and a great message – probably saved hundreds of lives. These people are heroes.

They are, and I had many an argument with the shill callers about them, one was so hot that I was kicked off a Telegram channel. It was an argument about Kate Shemirani, a former nurse who had her own megaphone and maybe an ego to boot but you needed that to have the balls to speak out. Some members of the group and the owner really disliked her (pathologically, IMHO) because she was seen with someone (rather, that someone was near her) who had been identified, by another someone, as being

77th Brigade – A UK forces counterintelligence psyop unit waging war against us. She was 'controlled opposition', a 'shill' they said. In my opinion, the shills could have been some of them, sowing divide and suspicion. My mantra was to look at what the individual is actually doing, is it net good or net bad? These heroes were losing their jobs and family and often their health, my admiration for them is immense. I had the same arguments about Musk and Trump. Although I was one of the first to join the group and had helped the owner access Truth Social even before it was available in the UK, I was booted off. I guess the clique system I encountered in some football teams runs the same in all groups. Shame. Never mind, I formed my own.

Back to London. An emotion was brewing. Kate and Delores spoke along with a few others, I had no idea what they said as I was behind them talking to an ex-paratrooper from Scotland. People came from all over, in groups or individually. The Police helicopters hovered above. This was a massive event, I was thinking to myself, this is going to make waves in the news – nothing has been this big.

Some fireworks went off and I could see people peeling off in the far-left corner, making their way up Whitehall, towards Downing Street. I tried to get around so I was somewhere in the middle of the carnival – that's what it felt like. I hardly saw any police, but they were at the sides and seemed to be in charge of where the route was to meander. I was just soaking it in, it really felt like the mafia had met their match. Deciding that I didn't want to be caught up in the mayhem of getting home with thousands of others, I decided to duck into a side street, after passing Downing

Street, and make my way home. The procession had a permanent bulge next to the Prime Minister's residence as there was an extra special party vibe generated, all kinds of offerings were being thrown, but it was peaceful. I ducked into Whitehall Place to take a breather and video the spectacle. I was surrounded by vans of Fuzz, police everywhere hiding, waiting to pounce – sneaky.

There was a permanent buzz of helicopters and a never-ending stream of protesters passing by.

I would estimate they were 30 – 50 people deep and the procession lasted 40 minutes to an hour to pass. It was phenomenal, hundreds of thousands. This was one massive event. It will change everything. I thought.

I reported back to my family, live whatsapping video, they must have been watching on the news, and they must be kicking themselves for not being involved.

Heading home, I texted my wife. 'What's it like on the news, what are they saying?'

'Can't see anything', 'nothing', they say there is a 'Free Palestine' march but otherwise nothing.

Now I saw that Free Palestine march, on my way there, it was tiny, about 100 people, but lots of police before and aft. Didn't think much of it.

'What, nothing about this???' 'it's fucking massive, nothing?' 'Nah, can't see anything'.

At that moment, I knew the mainstream media were going to be our biggest enemies, they are the Cabals' Goliaths.

On the train home, I scanned the news channels. I thought how great the day was yet realised I had only seen either people like me, awake and active, or the police, we didn't encounter one 'normie'.

Nobody saw anything on TV.

It suddenly dawned upon me that the whole thing was a complete waste of time. A big echo chamber event.

The next day a couple of news channels mentioned a few hundred 'anti-vaxers' – A few hundred! For the love of God!!!

Every so often, reality hits you. Has there ever been a time in history when the British people have been so attacked by their own 'government', the opposition, and the independent media? all together as one – against the people.

This - Is – exactly - what's – happening - right – now, I remind myself in utter disbelief.

How come this happens in my bloody lifetime, at my age?? My kids are too young to deal with it, my parents too old – no, it's all down to me! What are the odds of that happening? This cannot be simply down to chance, something out of this world is at play. Maybe it's time to find God.

Battle of the Band. Hyde Park.

I didn't go but there was a Jam for Freedom gathering organised for Hyde Park, later in the day.

This led to one of the most spectacular backfires in 'community policing' I have ever seen – it was as magnificent as it was horrifying.

Hyde Park, near 'Speakers Corner' – the home of free speech, the very symbol of the right to protest – it is what the United Kingdom stood for.

A beautiful spring evening.

The girl with the pink jumper was sat behind her drums, the tall guy with a grey hoodie was singing accompanied by an orange-haired mop-top guy in sunglasses. A keyboard stood alone, unmanned. It was sunset. A beautiful crisp evening in London. 'Don't look back in anger' was coming to its end, the crowd were happy, singing, arms aloft, big smiles, peacefully enjoying each other's company, they were as diverse as you wish, united in hope.

Harmless.

The people stood and sang 360 degrees around the musicians, no stage, very limited equipment, low volume but enough to start a sing-along. An hour before, the crowd was much larger, most had already set off home. It was winding down; a good day had been had.

The drummer brought the song to its end with a snare/floor tom fill and the inevitable splash of a cymbal. There were cheers of joy. Then the guitarist played the opening riff to 'Californication' with a fuzzy vibrato on his small practice amp. 'Yes, yes, play that one', a lady pleads, the singer was searching his phone for the lyrics, and the impromptu song started...

What happened next should be written into English folklore. A seminal moment. Watching it now makes my heart race like I am watching the last five minutes of an England rugby team fighting to win a World Cup final, could go either way. You sit, mouth open, barely breathing.

Groans, moans, and the boos, that was the first hint of something. Then the boos get louder as you see glimpses of yellow vests, Police hats and masks.

Barging their way towards the band, pushing people over so they fall back and under the advancing mob (Police). It was an unstoppable momentum they had created. Obviously, some bright spark in charge had led from the front, his minions lined up behind forcing their way into the inner circle. As those at the front met with the physical resistance of their innocent victims falling in front of them, their colleagues were still in full advance. This created one shove too many.

There were maybe 10 police officers in this first group, they looked utterly ridiculous in their masks, they weren't wielding batons, in fact, their arms were kind of pressed into their sides due to the pressure they created by forcing into a gap that wasn't there. So, they all fell into the drums, unable to stop themselves, on top of some poor souls who were peacefully singing 10 seconds before.

This has to be one of the most bungled police moves in history. What were they thinking? Who did they think they were? Who was trying to impress who? I suspect it was one male officer trying to impress a female officer behind him – look at me, look how brave I am, watch me deal with this. It was such a stupid act that it had to be on impulse for such a stupid reason. Unless this was planned – and if so, collective stupidity just hit a new low.

'Out, get out, go home NOW', one shouted

People snapped. What do you do if some idiot is pushing you hard into a drum kit? Drum Kits aren't made for comfort. You push back, you have to, otherwise, your ribs crack. This little push-back created an unstoppable counter energy, 15 minutes of glorious people power.

Fear in their eyes, masks puffing in and out quickly, Police looking back at their colleagues pleading for them to stop pushing. Maybe looking back in anger. 'Stop, stop - Back, go back, BAAAAACK!'.

The tide turned instantly. A few smoke bombs hit the scene. The retreat was clumsy, they were becoming surrounded. The image was of mayhem in smoke with a setting sun behind, like a picture of the battle of waterloo in oils. One female officer, for some inexplicable reason tried to pull back a drum in their retreat, like a teenager exiting a 'The Who' concert with a Keith Moon memento. Her hands were beaten off, she lost grip, and fell backwards, one of the crowd helped her up.

Bottles started to rain down, some with contents filling the skies, then a scooter, then fruit (pears, I believe). You can hear and see 2 or 3 members of the audience shouting 'stop', but it was too late. A sleeping giant had awoken, and he was somewhat 'pissed'.

The smoke bombs came in crimson and green; the light was a fantastic low and sharp sunset; the noise became a roar and somewhere a small amp was feedbacking. It was like the finale of an epic gig. Unforgettable.

There seemed to be two sets of retreating and exposed Police 'gangs', all walking backward, truncheons raised like cornered cobras. Fear in the eyes, pathetically shouting 'Get Back Now', the advancing crowd was in their faces – 'you get back', 'you're the violent ones', 'this is your fault' – 'you go home'.

'Back off' the Police shouted, 'You back off' came the reply. They did.

This had to be made clear, cameras were everywhere, 'This will be on YouTube, everyone will see what happened'. However, people also knew the deep-state players would take that down and all that would be left would be the body cam footage from the police, conveniently missing the first minute. It will look like they were attacked, and people will be arrested further down the line. The peaceful singers would be Far-Right Terrorists.

Ten minutes of retreat followed by more bottles raining down, screams of abuse, a loud constant rage. Police were walking backward but hitting out, some trying to grab people but failing. One of the Police groups took it to another level by attempting to fight back, this did not work, they became overwhelmed, many a hat was lost by this time, one officer had a bloody eye and was being shielded by a member of the audience, the numbers of people trying to quell the violence increased, they were trying to protect the officers.

Clearly, there was no plan B for this 'tactical' police operation. Immensely stupid. The noise and anger increased as more people joined the advance. The two Police groups managed to unite but they were still in full retreat, not turning their back to run (which may have been a better option) but holding onto each other briskly walking backward, eyes darting all over. Very scared. How much more foolish could they look, I don't know.

Eventually, they backed themselves onto a road to a chorus of 'Shame on you, shame on you', it appeared some reinforcements had arrived, but not a lot. They formed a line between barriers and a standoff ensued, abuse flying both ways. A full line of the crowd had linked arms in front of the Police to protect them – I suppose I'm right in thinking none of them were thanked, 'Do bears shit in the woods?' I hear you think.

Some calmness descended, probably due to a mutually felt exhaustion. Peace fizzled in.

Being a fly on the wall at the first debrief must have been like watching Sir Alex Ferguson giving his players the 'hairdryer' treatment, after a humiliating defeat where every single player forgot their lines.

"What the fuck were you doing?" If this wasn't the first thing said to the officer in charge, I will eat my hat.

Police thuggery of this nature has been widespread, particularly in Australia, The Netherlands, and Canada, it seems to happen very easily, it happens in all authoritarian regimes, this time though, people are armed, with cameras. Yes, a lot of them remove their badge numbers, and naturally, they are all masked but if you watch the video of this Hyde Park event, you will see many can, and will, be identified. ('Police chased out of Hyde Park after attacking peaceful protest' Rumble.com)

May 8th, 2021. Brighton.

My wife and I travelled to Brighton to attend a March for Freedom. A lot of our new friends were going and there would be plenty of Covid Marshals there, so it sounded fun. We were to meet at the Peace Statue, where some people would speak and then we would walk through town, the route seemingly unplanned so far. There were about 30 people there when we arrived and about 60 police officers in some kind of 'play it down', blue over-jackets, keeping the obligatory 'thumb-rester' holes. As with a lot of these demonstrations, there was a large contingent of hippie-looking types, and some were there just to create trouble (not sure at the time, but clearly agitators were placed there by the opposition). They were all nice and honest hippies, but probably didn't do our PR much good – we liked to think of ourselves as the owners of better science, and at least equally educated with our enemy. I guess what I'm saying is that some looked like tin foil hat wearers. I would later find myself defending such accusations on Twitter to be faced with images of protestors looking like tin foil hat wearers. It just made things more difficult when 'Red Pilling' what was already a Clown World. Piers Corbyn was an example, he was at all such events, a good guy with a strong scientific background, an Astrophysicist, but equally, he gave the opposition some ammo, just by the way he looked – it's shit, but that's how things work.

Within an hour our numbers had massively increased, the London contingent had arrived. The police and COVID marshals looked concerned but remained friendly. To my surprise, I became over-excited, out of control and found myself hating them and shouting accusations at them, again, "Nuremburg 2 is coming for you," everything pent up from London, everything I mislearned as a 13-year-old punk came out, we had our own band back then, The Non-Conformists, we sang about Police Oppression and getting banged up on SUS (a law allowing police stop, search and arrest if they suspect you being involved in crime) – we were never arrested and 'Police Oppression' didn't really happen in rural Devon, where the local newspaper headlines read ' Old lady loses her purse'.

I did calm and someone kindly gave me a batch of 'The White Rose' stickers, these were great black and white rectangular stickers that were non-digital memes of the time, brilliant and witty, they were everywhere. I remember they had a telegram channel with a feature that displayed their stickers from all corners of the globe – they deserve so much credit.

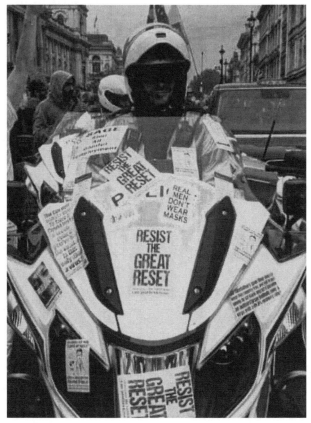

Someone gave a signal and we all marched off down the promenade towards the city centre. We probably stretched half a mile. Again, the sun was out, the Gods were on our side, and people from all walks of life and from all backgrounds.

As we walked through the city, we were flanked by the 'general public' and very few supported us, they were hurling abuse at us. 'Fuck off you idiots', 'nutters', 'you'll get us all killed, put your fucking masks on'. Wow, pure hatred. You couldn't hold a conversation with any of them, they just shouted insults. I just found myself shouting 'Take your fucking masks off.' I hated them back. Collaborators. It was heated and I felt like we were being paraded around the city to be made examples of, surprised we didn't end up in stocks in the town square.

We all stopped by the BBC offices, ten minutes later it was completely plastered in White Rose stickers, as was a shop 100% dedicated to Covid Masks, on the opposite side. Good.

Clot Shots

Once you've been screamed and shouted at, and called morons, by morons, you start to get a thicker skin. You find yourself making points and comments that could be inflammatory, as long as you know what you are talking about – believe me, the morons don't. They are highly emotional and ready to hurl insults but not facts. You become used to it, and you can offload your message with very little in return.

As soon as the vaccinators became visible in our cities, they would inevitably draw attention from those of us having to take direct action. The first ones I saw popped up on the public lawns, old ambulances, or portacabins, big signs stating 'NHS Vaccinations'. A whole city car park had also been tuned into a dedicated space with red signalling on the roads, there were queues leading into all of them, all day, every day. Approaching the temporary units, you would see signs saying, 'Protect your loved ones, get your vaccination here', or 'One in three people with Covid are asymptomatic'.

It would really wind me up, you knew it was bullshit propaganda.

The sheep were obeying.

I got my practice in spontaneously, you can't help it. Walking past them, before you know it, you've shouted 'IDIOTS', 'FOOLS'. I would also find myself walking really close to the line, holding my phone to my ear, nobody on the other end, loudly saying, 'Yeah, I know, fools all lined up, they've no idea it's poison'.

I would then find myself approaching the staff, the 'nurses' and security. 'Which vaccine are you doing today? 'Astra Zeneca', one and two', they would say proudly. 'Is that the one with the chimpanzee virus in it?' I would ask. 'Err, not sure really' they would giggle. 'Do you know what's in it?' I would ask, before giving them a chance I would then say, 'You don't do you?' 'And the people you are injecting don't know also', 'how can they give informed consent? 'You do know people are dying from these?' 'People who have a 99.9996% covid survival rate', 'You will be on the wrong side of history' – by now the security are standing around them, muttering 'ant-vaxers, anti-vaxers', and the nurses are sticking their fingers in their ears, 'not listening', 'not listening', 'thank you, bye bye'.

They had been briefed. I know because I stood in one briefing session once, they kept asking me to move back but I heard the mantra – do not engage!

The fact is, the vaccinators thought they were saving the world, they were heroes, probably the same heroes producing the dance videos six months beforehand. They really thought they were doing good and me coming in and talking to them like that very much pissed on their chips.

The more you do it, the better you get, but it is still nerve-wracking, especially if you are next to a bunch of customers who are high on their cognitive dissonance, relieved that their beloved authorities have come to save them. Many had been holed up way after lockdown, petrified that the latest viral mutation had their address and was waiting to pounce around the nearest corner. They had doubled up on the mask and braved the pandemic to get to receive the chance of life, they certainly won't entertain the thought of me taking that from them. For those, I was the bringer of certain death. There were others who believed in the efficacy of the shots so much that they needed theirs to protect their parents who had already had them but were 'vulnerable' – as the BBC told them.

There was a new bus, all brightly decorated and welcoming on the seafront. It soon attracted a steady queue, I had some of my 'informed consent' forms folded in my pocket so thought it a good idea to speak with the poor souls lining up for their pointless poison. At this point parents were bringing their 'over 12-year-olds', they were super keen. I had watched Dr Robert Malone, the inventor of mRNA technology, speak to parents directly about the risks and cribbed my key points from him.

I approached the line, barriers on either side just like the sheep dip it was. I imagined sometimes people halfway along may have thought about changing their decision, but turning back would create such a bother, they would ignore their intuition.

So, I started to talk at them.

Injecting your child is decision that is irreversible.

Here's some scientific facts about this genetic vaccine.

It is a viral gene that will be injected into your children's cells.

This gene forces your child's body to make toxic spike proteins.

These proteins can cause permanent damage in your children's organs their brain and nervous system. Their heart and blood vessels, creating blood clots.

Their reproductive system can be damaged, do you want to have grandchildren?

'Shut up mate, go away' 'we don't care what you say'

Their immune system will be damaged, and it will be irreparable.

This novel technology has not been fully tested. It's experimental! It normally takes five years to know if a medicine is safe. These won't be safe.

'We don't care' 'we don't care', They kept saying that to me, in front of their kids. The kids started to become abusive – they weren't even listening to what I was saying, they just hated me.

Your children represent no danger to their parents or grandparents. You get the jabs if you think they will protect you, if they protect you, why jab your kids?

'Fuck off mate'. Nobody took my leaflets. The vaccinators called the police. I didn't hang around for them but knew I was being filmed.

9. Serving Notice

I travelled back to Brighton to join in a demonstration against their massive, central shopping centre-based vaccine facility. This was constructed quickly within a very large but closed clothing outlet. My friend picked me up along the way, the sun was shining and Sweet Caroline by Niel Diamond came on the radio – we launched into a full-throated sing-along boosting our sympathetic nervous systems ready to fight (no flight intended).

When we got there, we saw plenty of Police near the doors, people were going in at a steady stream and coming out 'Team Pfizer' proud. There were maybe 20 of us, some had useful flyers a few had placards. We spoke with people as they entered, most barged past hurling insults but some stopped, some listened, and some turned away, often with children. Some people clearly wanted to know more about our information, doubts were starting to creep in.

Then our side numbers grew, significantly. Again, groups from London and Kent, turned up, some very vocal and a few aggressively vocal, things started to feel a bit off. I was smashed into by a vaccine customer, a tall and fat bloke who was clearly angry with the world. He didn't fancy a chat. Another customer, a 'more than middle-aged' lady came right up to me, face in mine, 'my Mum died of Covid, what you are doing is criminal', 'You are just conspiracy theorists – brainwashed'. *'Sorry to hear of your loss, but how do you know it was Covid?'* 'Hospital told me', 'It was Covid, you lot are mad, you're evil'. Judging by her age, her mother must have been in her nineties.

Then Kate Shemirani arrived, with her megaphone. All I knew about her was that she used to be a fairly senior nurse, had survived cancer, and knew all the granular biology and chemistry around the 'faults' in the PCR tests and mRNA jabs. She had spoken in London and seemed to deal with aggressive normies with better wordplay than them, she would ask them questions and they would wilt immediately. She is a powerhouse. Also there, was Anna de Buisseret, a lawyer with a military background. She is also a force to be reckoned with – although currently fighting her own health battles, prayers going her way. She knew the law and she knew how to inform the vaccinators they were committing crimes. She managed to gain entry, stick her megaphone inside the doors and effectively serve notice to all inside. Once served notice the jab givers could not plead ignorance in the future. Both Kate and Anna, took things to a new level that day. The centre closed until everyone dispersed, someone set a firework off, giving the press that extra bit of juice to accuse us of firebombing the building, effectively setting us up as domestic terrorists. All rouge governments around the world call their opposition terrorists. It's that old Marxist tactic.

The Child Catcher

Walking back from the shops one day I saw this poster. I stopped, looked, rubbed my eyes, looked again, and could not believe what I was seeing. This has to be a joke, surely?? It wasn't, they were really planning this – for families, for the kids. FREE FUN DAY – WITH VACCINES......!!!

A free fun day for the family and the top attraction was a 'no booking required' Vaccine bus!!!

Holy shit, how sinister, how low have things sunk?

I instantly thought of, by far, the scariest film character ever, The Child Catcher, from Chitty Chitty Bang Bang, a terrifying, evil nightmare of a character. He still scares the crap out of me.

This was it, this was their cunning plan now, 'entice the little fuckers out with sweets and jab them'.

I had to get this stopped.

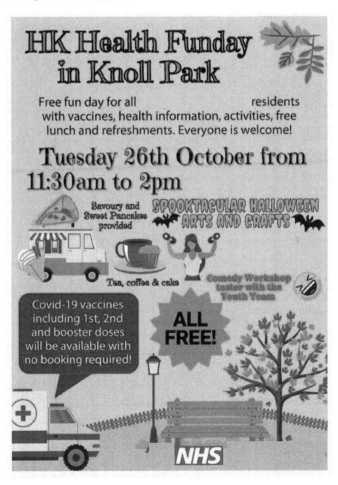

I passed a picture of the poster around Telegram, some people responded with a crying/laughing emoji, obviously thinking it was a joke. I have redacted some of the names, but one, the fitness project, was a company owned by a friend, a very awake friend. He was gobsmacked that someone from his team thought this was a good idea – associating themselves with this monstrosity of an event – apparently, they were committed with participants and couldn't find a way out of it.

People came back to me, is this really happening? They said, 'Oh my god, we have to stop it. Word got out very quickly, we were going to meet at 11 am, with the aim to try and intercept the vax bus, there were two ways in and out for vehicles, so we would divide when there. As I was driving near the small park, I noticed Police vans everywhere, mainly around both entrances, I continued driving and informed the channels we were communicating on. I parked some distance away, grabbed my flyers and burner phone, leaving my main mobile in the car. We had been infiltrated; the Police obviously knew we were coming.

Around six of us were there first, the Police asked us why we were there, we were clear, we had come to persuade parents not to jab their children. They were non-threatening, and a couple also allowed themselves to look at our literature.

'You're wasting your time here though, no vaccines going on here today', one said.

We found out they had cancelled the Vax Bus, they told us, 'It ain't coming, we knew you lot would turn up', they didn't want any violence in front of children – apparently. 'Violence?', moi? Isn't jabbing children violent?

So, the fun day was just pancakes, arts and crafts, and a fitness demo – rubbish really, we felt like party poopers. Just as soon as we were told this, a large army of protesters from Kent arrived, maybe twenty of them led by a couple of well-known, self-proclaimed, leaders in the 'freedom movement'. Our numbers from the local area rose to around the same – so, forty or fifty of us in total, about 15 local residents, including a few bored kids, and maybe 20 Police. It was highly unbalanced.

We were standing at one end of the field the police encircled around the people not having fun at the fun day. The Kent lot decided to spread out in a line, unfurling banners, and started shouting at the fun seekers. The fun seekers started shouting back, one of whom was my neighbour. She didn't notice me, but she was usually a sweet mild-mannered lady, until now – she was bright red in rage, literally spitting as she was shouting, calling all the banner holders c*nts. It was a complete farce, some people travelled well over an hour to get there, but we were happy that no child got jabbed – that was all that mattered. Yes, we would have liked to have rolled the Vax Bus on its side and chased the jabbers out of the park. I, personally, was going to track down, and slay the Child Catcher – stake through the heart after a flurry of punches to the face and his stupid nose.

No Violence.

BTW, if you know who Jamie Raskin is, don't you think he is the spitting image of the Child Catcher?

In fact, to digress, why are the lying, cheating, corrupt deep-state players so ugly? They are! They all really look evil. Why can't the normies see this??

The child catcher missed his opportunity on this occasion, but his success rate is becoming very clear. As I type, the CDC are being forced to release some dreadful statistics.

A 'fact-checked' report by 'The Peoples Voice' states:

'The official figures reveal that there was a slight increase in excess deaths among children and young adults when the alleged Covid pandemic hit the U.S. in early 2020.

However, with the introduction of a Covid injection, one would have expected deaths to have fallen significantly among the age group in 2021.

Instead, however, the opposite happened.

Excess deaths among children and young adults were significantly higher every single week in 2021 than they were in 2020 except for weeks 29 and 30.

But then in week 31, something drastic happened to cause excess deaths to skyrocket among children and young adults.

And official figures provided by the CDC, unfortunately, show that trend has continued in 2022.

The most recent data released by the CDC covers up to week 40, the week ending October 9th, and it should be noted that the last few weeks of data are subject to change.

But 2022 has also been a significant year for excess deaths among children and young adults.

The CDC has confirmed that there have been 7,680 more excess deaths among children and young adults in 2022 so far than there were during the same time frame in 2020 at the height of the Covid pandemic.

The year 2021, was by and far the worst, however, with 27,227 more excess deaths by week 40 following the roll-out of the Covid-19 injection than what occurred in 2020 at the height of the pandemic.

But the most concerning figures reveal that the overall number of deaths and excess deaths among children and young adults spiked since the roll-out of the Covid injections.

Nearly half a million people aged 0 to 44 have sadly died since week 51 of 2020.

This has resulted in an astonishing 117,719 excess deaths against the 2015-2019 five-year average.'

Now, we hear the installed government in Brazil has made it a mandatory vaccination for children at school, the parents can opt-out, but then they don't get any financial welfare.

The Child Catcher is real.

-6029679/21

I was waiting for the others to show up, a demonstration had been planned to arrive at the new major vaccine jabbing event at a major sporting facility on the south coast. It was huge, the car park was full, a lot of people in yellow Hi-Viz's, pointing and marshalling.

Around twenty of us were going to form a line and hold placards up, handing out leaflets. We would be as welcome as a wasp in a tent.

I had been following events elsewhere, where it seemed some good progress was being made legally. Mark Sexton, a former police officer had started to formally report the Covid vaccination program to the police as a crime. And, so he should, we all should be. Clearly, something was very wrong where manufactured inaccuracies in case number reporting led to the widespread, mandated, injecting of untested, experimental concoctions into the arms of the uninformed public, it simply had to be a crime. Either a mass crime against humanity, breaking all Nuremberg Codes, or, at best, criminal negligence. Mark, along with a few others had bravely arranged an audience with senior police inspectors at various Police Stations, Including Hammersmith, in London.

He reported the crime and obtained a crime number: 6029679/21 – later to be disputed, but nevertheless, a seminal moment. Something tangible.

He had the support of lawyers, Philip Hyland and Lois Bayliss amongst others. These very brave souls had overridden obvious pressure to avoid the inevitable attack from 360 degrees, their families probably pleading with them to not get involved, their peers watching them commit career suicide (and helping). They took this 'apparent' crime very seriously – as lawyers should - and produced a framework for all of us to fall back on.

There were thousands of us, worldwide, going into vaccination centres, schools, and police stations to complain about their acquiescence, and collaboration, not to mention the direct lethally criminal actions of the vaccinators. Thousands of us relying on our own wits to deliver our message in a coherent, succinct, and sane manner, in the face of aggressive resistance.

At the end of the day, the crime number may be disputed as irrelevant by the Police, they started to say it was not, in fact, a crime number but simply a reference number to a conversation. Mark Sexton recorded his encounters, there is no disputing a crime was reported and that leaves the police with the heavy burden of having the ball firmly in their court when the full facts emerge, and they will, in fact, they are.

A lot of people are carrying that weight.

Why? Because they have been officially served notice. They have been handed their proof of guilt.

They knowingly continued to commit a crime. A crime they can no longer say they were not aware of.

I decided to bring a letter from one of the lawyers, designed to be a 'cease and desist' notice. Also, I had a well-thought-out information sheet, as used by Mark Sexton and countless others. I was never really that keen on 'protesting' in groups. I found the lack of control worrying, having no idea what someone would shout or do. The legitimacy and credibility of a protest can be easily undone with one stupid comment. Sometimes, our side looked a bit too hippy-ish – even though they are good people with noble intentions and brave actions, I feel bad saying so, but sometimes it is all about perception. If we were to change the opinions and behaviours of our fellow citizens, I felt we couldn't risk being dismissed as crazies. That was always the accusation –

anti-vaxxer loonies.

The lawyer's involvement and serious letter of notice was a game changer. It gave me confidence and I could clearly see the same effect, with thousands of others. Videos were appearing daily of people walking into vax centres, schools, police etc, and having the bravery to confront them with an official letter of notice – this tool was so powerful.

One thing I noticed in nearly all of the videos was that, in general, one person was the key talker, that person managed to grab the attention of the target. That person would be effectively communicating the message. Keep it succinct and simple. Deliver the message, hand over the letter politely, and exit. Job done.

What tended to happen was, other people around the main speaker would suddenly find some courage and 'pipe-up', they would talk over the main speaker, they would raise their voices and get angry, they would make the main speaker lose their rhythm and organised delivery, they would raise the ante and completely ruin the exercise. In short, they would 'play to the cameras'.

As I sat there, in my car, 'waiting for the mob' – seriously, no disrespect to any of you, you are all heroes – I started to think, if I'm going to do this, I should just go in now. Partly because, I felt if I had an audience behind me, the pressure to deliver would go up and my social anxiety would kick in.

I had to do it now – or probably not at all.

So, grabbing my folder of paperwork and my phone, I walked into the main foyer, it was full of people in their allocated waiting areas, all ages, by this time they were jabbing 5 – 11-year-olds, so there were plenty of parents and kids.

I set my phone camera to record and approached the main desk, this is the exact audio.

"Hello."

"Hello, are you booked in?"

"No, I want to show you this letter from lawyers acting to protect the public, you can give them a call to verify…"

"Ok let me pass you on to…"

"Yes, please find me someone senior, thank you."

A worried-looking chap came out

"Hi there."

"Hello there, um, I"m just handing this to you. It's a letter from some senior lawyers."

"Yeah."

"Um, you can verify it by calling them, essentially this is just to let you know that there is a live Police, criminal investigation into the Covid injection roll-out and there are batches in existence that are known to be killing people – now. I would strongly advise you to call them and they're advising you, strongly, to stop what you are doing because, if you know what's going on, you're going to implicate yourselves. There are medications that are proven to treat any variations of Covid at the moment, um, there's a live criminal investigation…"

"Can I just stop you there, I need to go and get another group of people."

"Absolutely yeah yeah yeah."

"Just wait there."

"Ok."

Two masked seniors came quickly, one a female nurse who

seemed fairly happy to engage and one male looking more administrative who looked petrified.

"Hi, so, I'd like to pass this onto you. It really is for your benefit. There is a live criminal investigation going on with Hammersmith Police. These lawyers, (waving the lawyer's letter) are working with them and you can phone them to verify them. A strong advice is that you stop doing anything right now because there are batches out there that are killing people, that is what we know. You cannot give anyone the ability to give informed consent if you don't know what vaccines you have got. It's very simple, it's a two-pager. It's to protect you, honestly. Just to let you know (the viewer) I'm handing this over."

"Ok, I'll um forward this to our legal team, so thank you," said the nurse eagerly walking off, scared boy following, hands in pockets.

"Ok, but I would make that call to them. Because the thing is, you're going to be liable if you, if you carry on doing what you're doing in the knowledge that there's some serious investigations taking place, OK? Thank you very much. Bye." They had disappeared around the corner before I'd finished.

I could hear people behind me muttering and groaning throughout, but also some people standing nearer so they could hear, and, for sure, some parents left the building with their kids un-jabbed.

The letter of notice
FOA: ALL VACCINATION CENTRES / HUBS ALL DOCTORS, NURSES, CLINICAL STAFF ANYONE ADMINISTERING OR CAUSING TO BE ADMINISTERED SARS-COV-2 VACCINATIONS

4th February 2022

Dear Sir/Madam

Immunisation SARS-COV-2 Injections

I write in connection with ANY proposed immunisation service that you might be inclined to provide, either directly or indirectly.

As you will be aware whilst caring for patients you have signed an oath: FIRST DO NO HARM!

You owe a legal obligation to each patient in your care.

We ask that you do the following:

1. Write to the CQC/ LMC /MHRA /GMC / RCN / NHS / JCVI / Rt Hon Sajid Javid and any

other relevant authority and inform them that the vaccination programme you are involved in

must be cancelled and the reason for cancellation is that the SARS- CoV-2 injections are under

police investigation.

Should you fail to write to them and assist in the cancellation of the immunisation sessions you will render yourself liable for any losses sustained as a result of the visit and liability could include criminal liability.

Informed consent is impossible to obtain as you are not:

1. Informing the patient that the roll out of the SARS-COV-2 injections are under Police investigation pursuant to crime reference number: 6029679/21. Most people, if given that information, would decline to give consent for treatment. Please ensure this letter is communicated to all patients.

2. Part of the Police investigation revolves around the alleged unlawful suppression of alternative treatments which have a far better safety profile. Informed consent is not possible if there is no discussion around safer alternatives.

3. Informing the patient of how much active ingredient is in each vial. The amount of active ingredient in each vial varies and it is a matter of public record that some batches kill and maim disproportionately. Witness statements will be considered by the Police from bad batch victims.

By way of example, one of them is now infertile, others have been suffering with mobility and paralysis of the face and limbs and many others are suffering from serious heart conditions such as myocarditis/pericarditis/myopericarditis. These people have medical evidence which states that the injection caused the infertility, immobility, paralysis, and heart conditions.

It is a fact that they received bad batches.

As informed consent is impossible to obtain, anyone injected on site has suffered a battery, regardless of any injury sustained.

Can you come back to me confirming that the immunisation programme you are involved in has been cancelled.

Yours faithfully

The info sheet
25 Feb 2022

To medical/health practitioners or staff, or those dealing directly/indirectly with vaccines,

We, and countless millions worldwide, have serious concerns regarding the safety of the Covid vaccines, as do many thousands of highly qualified doctors, nurses, health professionals, and scientists.

From 9 Dec 2020 to 9 Feb 2022, 1,458,428 suspected UK adverse drug reactions (ADRs) were reported by 445,256 people in the context of Covid vaccines, within the "Yellow Card" reporting system. 2,017 deaths were reported. Yellow Card reports don't prove the vaccine was the cause, however it's possible a significant or high percentage of the ADRs and deaths were caused by the vaccine.

It's estimated only 10% of serious ADRs are reported. If we assume 7% of the 1,458,428 suspected ADRs were "serious," that is 102,089 serious ADRs. Adjusting for underreporting, that becomes 1,020,890 serious ADRs.

Several "time vs death rate" charts indicate strong correlation between start of vaccine rollout and increased death rates. The correlation doesn't prove the vaccines are the cause, however they may be. The correlation adds another data point to a growing list.

People who have suffered Covid vaccine injuries, and in some cases death:

https://nomoresilence.world/series/uk/

https://needlebar.co.uk/the-stories/

https://www.realnotrare.com/realstories/tags/united-kingdom

https://www.covidvaccineinjuries.com/covid-vaccine-stories/

https://www.covidvaccineinjuries.com/twitter-feed/

https://www.covidvaccineinjuries.com/current-data/

https://www.covidvaccineinjuries.com/covid-vaccine-memorial-wall/

The pages above will show only a small fraction of those affected.

It is shocking, and cynical, that life-changing vaccine injuries experienced by many have attracted no media coverage whatsoever. This is corrupt beyond measure and should be of deep concern to all.

A crime was reported with Hammersmith Metropolitan Police CID, relating to the Covid vaccines. Over 400 statements, several from GPs, and many from those whose health has been impacted or severely impacted, were submitted. Some of the statements are from families of the deceased. The evidence includes testimony from NHS and care home whistleblowers, over 1000 scientific studies, and testimony of many renowned scientific/medical practitioners. Two independent forensic reports exposing harmful ingredients, eg graphene and glass shards, were submitted. A letter to Medicines and Healthcare products Regulatory Agency (MHRA) includes a summary of the evidence: https://pjhlaw. co.uk/wp-content/uploads/2021/12/letterMHRA.pdf

Although there appears to be resistance from the police to becoming involved, they cannot simply refuse to examine a large body of credible evidence if they are undertaking their duties and acting according to their oath, so ignoring the evidence may suggest malfeasance and/or dereliction of duty.

On 22 Oct 2020, Steve Anderson gave a presentation which included this draft list of possible adverse events:

Guillain-Barré syndrome, Acute disseminated encephalomyelitis, Transverse myelitis, Encephalitis / myelitis / encephalomyelitis / meningoencephalitis / meningitis / encepholapathy, Convulsions / seizures, Stroke, Narcolepsy and cataplexy, Anaphylaxis, Acute myocardial infarction, Myocarditis / pericarditis, Autoimmune disease, Deaths, Pregnancy and birth outcomes, Other acute demyelinating diseases, Non-anaphylactic allergic reactions, Thrombocytopenia, Disseminated intravascular coagulation, Venous thromboembolism, Arthritis and arthralgia/joint pain, Kawasaki disease, Multisystem Inflammatory Syndrome in Children, Vaccine enhanced disease.

It's questionable how a vaccine with that list was approved. However, that list wasn't included on Pfizer fact sheets, or discussed with people receiving the vaccine. More complete fact sheets were released in Jan 2022.

We urge all people to take personal responsibility for their actions. We have a collective duty to know whether the orders we follow truly represent the interests of the public. Following orders without question has been responsible for some of the worst atrocities observed in history. If our civilised society and education system has one benefit, it should be the ability to look to past mistakes and avoid repeating them.

A key principle of the UNESCO Universal Declaration of Bioethics and Human Rights 2005 is Article 6, covering

"Informed consent," meaning the person concerned must be given adequate information that they understand. Growing evidence of the risk of adverse events or death suggests that this principle is not being adhered to, which has crime implications. The issues mentioned with the Pfizer fact sheets further affect informed consent, as does the lack of explaining therapeutics and alternative treatments.

Substantial and steadily growing evidence points towards the SARS-CoV-2 vaccines causing harm. We urge all parties to cease administering the vaccines. People who continue to administer the vaccines, or directly/indirectly facilitate the continuing administering of the vaccines, could potentially be found guilty of one or more crimes.

People underestimating the seriousness of the events unfolding may be surprised when the full extent of what has taken place during Covid gradually becomes known. We urge people to practice critical thinking, and question whether the many "fact check" pages might be driven by motives/interests that are not aligned with the greater public good. The same applies to the many social media influences that seek to discredit those highlighting the harm that has resulted from the vaccines.

In addition to the legal implications, we hope people have a sense of moral obligation to act in ways that put the interest *of the public first. We believe that doing so necessitates the cessation of the Covid vaccine program.*

Please read the enclosed documents, and share this letter and those documents with colleagues, health/medicine practitioners, police officers, solicitors, and MPs, using links below.

Thank you for your time and attention,

Concerned citizens and residents of the United Kingdom

I sent the video to the lawyers and confirmed they had taken the letter. One small job done. I suppose one day that will lead to some justice.

Yellow Boarding

Another very effective tool was organised by a group known as 'Stand in the Park', at least, that is where I first heard of it. There were many other groups using it and it probably originated in another country – Canada maybe. However, Yellow boarding was a thing. It was happening in most towns and cities, a huge amount of people got involved and eventually, it amalgamated with 'outreach' events in city centres, attempts to just go out there, get amongst the people and offer information. I only did the yellow board events, they were fun.

A message was delivered in a series of yellow boards held up sequentially alongside a busy road, near a roundabout or junction, where the travellers would slow enough to read or even have to stop.

As an example:

DID YOU KNOW - 200 metres from the junction.

YOUR CHILDREN - 160m

HAVE ZERO RISK FROM COVID -120m

THEY ARE MORE LIKELY TO BE HARMED - 80m

BY THE JABS - 60m

1,400 DEATHS SO FAR FROM VACCINES - 40m

CLOTS, HEART ATTACKS, STROKES, CANCER - 20m

COVID IS A HOAX - 10 metres.

CASE NUMBERS ARE FAKE - At the traffic lights, at this point, leaflets were handed out.

Or better still a copy of 'The Light' Newspaper – a brilliantly researched monthly publication.

It was a fantastic gauge as to the 'feel of the nation' because supporters of the message would beep their horns, and the normies would either ignore with faces of disgust, or shout abuse. The favourite was always the 'wanker' hand sign. In the early days, it was expected of the white van workers coming home from a hard day's slog, they would impress their buddies with it – often shouting 'wankers' at the same time. I loved that because they failed to notice they had to stop right next to the yellow boarders at the lights – I would often choose that spot so I could laugh at them squirming. It must have seemed such a good idea just 30 seconds back.

The first one I did was at a busy roundabout with traffic lights just before, so a great place for traffic congestion. You had to pick the right level of congestion, too much and the commuters were just pissed off, they would have no time for you, and you would just be a great 'stress offloading' target.

Enough congestion for the messages to be read. This was early

2021. We received around 1 beep per 20 cars – around 8 in 20 hurled insults, most ignored but you would get a lot of patronising shaking of the heads in fierce disapproval. I only did four and the last one was around October 2021. This time we were hitting a good 6 in 20 beeps and much less abuse, a few thumbs up.

Then the police turned up and thought it a good idea to speak with us one by one, walking along the line. As they approached, I thought it a good time to switch my phone camera on.

"Hello, how are you today sir," said the copper with his mask under his moustache yet above his mouth – impressive, I thought.

"I'm good, thanks."

"Were just having a double check making sure that everything's all right," he said. "Just been down on the London Road. I think there's a similar group to you, with a few people who have been beeping (he had to raise his voice over the support we were getting) but also people being not so nice, so we just wanted to check you are alright, really."

"Oh, thank you," I said, genuinely, as a one of his fully masked colleagues maneuvererd himself into position.

"All good. Yeah, thanks for that."

"Is it all good," he asked as his body cam red flashed itself as the big giveaway. "It's stopped raining for you here also, so that's nice," he said as I dropped my shades down over my eyes and pulled my hat lower.

"Yes, it's lovely now, thank you for your concern."

His buddy then stepped in, "I, I, I, don't know if there's a link to your group or anything but another group on er, er ,er, London Road area with similar signs, and there were a few er, er , er people being a bit unpleasant about it and ob, ob, obviously we want to ensure people conduct themselves in a lawful manner'" he said, red light flashing like mad. So, we want to be here to make sure there is no breach of the peace occurring and can help as far as we can be to er, to er, help with that," wringing his hands profusely.

"Thank you very much," I said looking way off to my right.

"Are you planning to be here about half hour longer, or, or...?"

"Yup, I've gotta go in about twenty minutes or so."

"Ok lovely," they said as they moved on to a colleague.

For the record, both officers were polite and clearly had a job to do. I would imagine their facial recognition technology can cope with sunglasses and hats, so they must have me filed away and labelled as Public Enemy Number One-hundred and twenty-seven-thousand, two-hundred and sixty-three. No doubt I'm in the 'Far-Right terrorist' category.

Digital Soldier / Keyboard Warrior

In October 2022, Elon Musk forced the sale of Twitter. It was an audacious move and brilliantly executed. Twitter was the hub for the deep state, they set it up as a place to mould thought. To trick people into thinking what they wanted them to think, to give the false impression that the majority have views that were the right views. The social engineering algorithm department was probably a relatively small one, a few people controlling so many – The wizard behind the curtain. The criminal mafia communicated in the back channels with each other, it was their plaything. Like Google, Twitter was a tool to influence voters. If you use Google now and don't see the blatant hard-left bias, you are either so hard-left it feels normal, or you are as intelligent as an amoeba.

Single cellular.

Twitter was used to label anyone with a slight right leaning of being Far-Right and, therefore racist. Homophobic and all the others. You were THE cause of all human misery; you were led to believe you had thoughts that should section you under the Mental Health Act. Thoughts that you may just want to pull far-left ideology, slightly right and back towards the middle, just slightly – there you go, Racist, Far-Right, Far-Right but still left of centre. This is what they did.

Put it this way, if you were a mild-mannered simple guy with no political leanings other than to live and let live, you could coast along quite happily. Then you may start to think about things, how society could be organised, you may develop ideas yourself or start to study the philosophies and politics of others. If, as a metaphor, you were happily travelling up the Greenwich meridian with your simple 'middle of the road' politics and you took a left turn, heading west, as you started to think socialist, you may find yourself in North America. If you became a little more radical, you would go further left heading west to Hawaii, by which time you may be a little Marxist. If you keep going, becoming harder and harder towards communism and totalitarianism, you would travel further left, further west, to the point you have reached Hong Kong. Now you have found yourself in the Far East – Far Right – you Fascist pig!

Talking communism, it was a well-known plan that America could be overrun and turned into a communist state by stealth, without a bullet being fired. A slow infiltration of behaviour, ideas, and social engineering. Look at TikTok in the West, how it encourages self-indulgence, fragile egos, victim mentalities, body shaming, trans ideology, weakness, the notion of hate, and the spread of 'isms. In China, TikTok for the kids is more for showing achievement, excellence, mathematic genius, musical maestros, and sporting success. The West takes its new values into its armed forces, we have generals in lipstick. If we went to war with China, just pure 'man on man' fighting, who would win?

Football

That brings me to football. Oh dear. Such role models they are, a slight brush of a hand near the face and they go down like a sniper was in the stands. Rolling around patting their moisturised faces looking for blood, medical teams rushing on-field holding their head and neck in a firm neutral position for fear of instant paralysis. I mean they should be a little more vocal and concerned about the ones keeling over with vax-induced heart attacks, but alas not.

Imagine you are an old-school football manager, a Mike Bassett, as some in the UK will know. Imagine trying to set your warriors up for battle, you explain the tactics, positions and set pieces, then time for the rousing speech. You fire them up, they will die for you and the team, fight till the bitter end, 'who dares wins' SAS mentality, victorious glory awaits...

Then they line up and hold the hand of a small child, cameras in their faces, bend down and speak with the child extruding energies of kindness. They walk out into the arena and stand in a line, they sing a song about the King living long before they walk along to face their enemy and shake their hands, maybe a cuddle. They may exchange gifts to each other. Then, because someone has died, anyone, the kit man's ex-lover, they stand in a circle and bow their heads, deeply emotional – if you're lucky, they include the mascot, now that is funny as funny can be, a line of solemn mourners, heads bowed, then a big gormless grin from ear to ear from a fat-headed goose, priceless comedy - they may clap facing each other for a minute, then the whistle blows and they jump up and down for 30 seconds before taking their positions. The captain sets his rainbow armband in a comfortable place before they all take the knee. Ukrainian flags mingle with rainbow flags, everyone claps the knee pose. The virtueometer explodes.

I imagine that rousing team talk to fire them up for battle is a distant memory, they are probably all reduced to tears and wobbly legs, some war cry – it's hardly the bloody Haka is it!

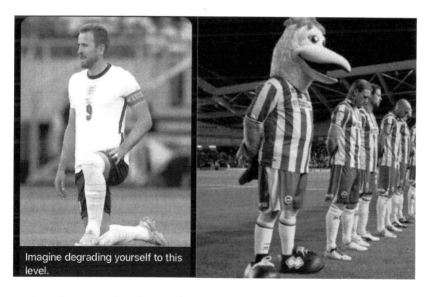

Imagine degrading yourself to this level.

Google, Facebook, and Twitter were all spreading such 'approved' thought. On the surface, seemingly benign, but, in fact, dangerous social and psychological weapons.

The deep state-owned it along with all mainstream media. With such blanket control, we had no hope.

Musk brilliantly used the laws protecting shareholders to force the sale. Stupidly, the deep state allowed Twitter to look like a fair and open company, they got complacent and that was their downfall, shareholders just wanted profit, Musk offered that. At this point, I will add that I believe Musk to be a White Hat player, a key player with a history of 'optics', and may well be in team Q.

I became a second-wave Anon, looking for comms, deciphering, linking to posts, and making sense of recent events with the information in the posts. I have been doing this since late 2021. Post 4511 June 24th, 2020, states, 'this has never been attempted' and goes on to explain the Military/Civilian alliance that is the essence of Q. People would annoyingly say that us 'Qtards' were just sitting back, waiting to be saved – no, far from it, we had a lot of work to do. We had to keep the message going, keep informing people that the plan was unfurling, stop people from clinging to dates, we had to curb our own enthusiasm for dates and predictions, and we sometimes let that slip. We had to keep spirits up and try to give people hope, based on the messages we were getting.

The new, and free Twitter allowed us to do this, anons could communicate and share reasoned debate over anything debatable, but in general, we all agreed pretty quickly. Twitter allowed a million digital soldiers and keyboard warriors – a Musk / Q alliance in my opinion.

I have written about this in one of the Substacks but have to say this takeover was a fundamental moment in the fightback, probably essential for its success.

Twitter became the new battleground for me.

I had a lot going on, on Telegram, but that was another echo chamber, in fact, I soon created a Telegram group specifically to create written 'ammo' for Twitter.

For the first time, we can actively call out the cabal and their minions, the scientists, doctors, reporters, and politicians, we can prove them to be liars, expose the cheats, correct their bad science, challenge their biased reporting, and publicly accuse them of crimes against humanity. A great hashtag was the 'never forget' label we could attach to those in the public eye who called for the punishment of the unvaccinated. They will not ever be allowed to excuse themselves, no amnesty, the storm is coming (for them).

Musk entered his new offices carrying a kitchen sink. Only those who know Q know what that means.

He is also the provider of Starlink, an internet system that cannot be turned off by the deep state. Starlink and US Space Force have an alliance that, in my humble opinion, will bite the asses of the Cabal. Sometime soon, in a way that will scupper one of their false flag blackout plans to stop the next US election.

The humour and intelligence in Musk's counter-offensive is hugely entertaining. Take his new AI tool Grok. Designed to counter the ChatGPT AI system everyone is starting to play with. ChatGPT, has an obvious left bias to it, it is clearly the next level Google, an influencer, a thought manipulator, social engineering.

Grok, on the other hand, has been tweaked to be sarcastic and rebellious! Brilliant! But for what purpose? How does that help?

Well, it serves to show us all that AI is not the future, it is not something to rely on, it's only as good as the programmers behind it. If those programmers are baddies, we are toast.

That is exactly why Grok is 'sarcastic', it's to show AI could also be 'evil'.

Genius.

10. My Long Vax Syndrome – Getting Stoned in Jericho

This is a two-for-one deal. You get the Israeli-Palestinian experience bundled in with the inoculation soup story, resulting in a case of Long Covid – or whatever its ancestor was called in the Eighties. It's a family bumper pack deal of the century, hurry while stocks last.

Yellow Fever, Hepatitis A & B, Typhoid, Rabies, Polio Booster, Meningitis, Diphtheria, Pertussis, Tetanus, Varicella, and Pneumococcus – take your pick. I had a bundle, a soup, all injected in me the same day. It was the Eighties so I have no idea what the soup ingredients contained but it would have been several of the above. I was travelling to Israel. No particular reason other than it was as far away from a Technical College in Devon that me and my mate had slumbered in for two years, in fact I hardly went, such was my enthusiasm for clearly the absolute worst choice in studies. Let's go somewhere mental, completely alien – how about a war zone, one of us said.

My friend made bombs. Word would get out at school, Matt's doing a bomb tonight, 10 pm, River Beach. He would keep his build spec secret, but I was pretty sure it involved drainpipes (as I saw him exiting the plumbers' merchants), weedkiller, and sugar. Secretly, he would be down there in the dark, with his spade and explosives digging deep into the sand, preparing the show. Bizarrely, nobody really saw him arrive, do his deed, or leave, yet at 10 pm sharp in an area naturally cordoned off by boats, netting, and a jetty, there was the mother of all BOOMS. Deep vibrations felt under your feet, a thud of heavy dub bass in your chest, and a sound like you were within thunder. Bloody brilliant.

Sixteen years before, there was the Six-Day War, Israel had captured the Golan Heights from Syria, The West Bank of East Jerusalem, The Gaza Strip, and the Sinai Peninsula from Egypt. A long time beforehand but obviously still very hot.

At this point, it's best to say, I, and we, had no ties, connections of sympathies with either side, and still don't. We were still teenagers and had no idea of the histories or cultures, we just smoked pot, played in a punk band, and did some art.

Anyway, one of us heard that you could get free accommodation for as long as you like, if you didn't mind picking Avocados in the mornings somewhere near the Sea of Galilee, or Masada, The Dead Sea, Jerusalem, or Bethlehem – all sounded awesome. You get days off and free excursions to crazy places you only heard of in religious education, which, for me, was a made-up fantasy land. You can party for the rest of the day and night and there's bound to be exotic chicks from exotic places, plus they had Arak – a legendary and potent 'spirit of the anise family' (sounds so cute).

Kibbutz.

We made our way to the office of the organisers in London to find out where we would be posted, I hoped somewhere south near the coral beaches of the Red Sea, I had also heard the far north is still volatile, lots of live ammunition everywhere, guns and the occasional rocket attack. And cold.

We were allocated the most northern kibbutz possible, right next to the borders of Lebanon and Syria. They showed us images of the guns we would encounter and maps of the currently live minefields that were literally surrounding us, and pictures of the explosive material we would find littering the whole Golan Heights area. They also liked to bus us in at night under armed guard.

Not the beach then.

Matt wore a strange smile.

A short while before leaving, I went to get my shots, I had several. As I go on to say, I have no idea what, but it seemed the 'better safe than sorry' logic was applied in my case as Matt only had one – maybe because he had previously travelled somewhere long haul a few months before with his parents.

My arm hurt like hell the next day. When I got up from bed I wobbled and felt sick. My vision and head were like the worst hangover I had experienced but I had a sober night. When I spoke, there was a weird echo. There was a strange 'buzz' going through me like someone had 'slipped me a Mickey'- spiked, drugged. I felt like I was in another body. I felt strangely depressed – was always happy-go-lucky but just felt down, very low, and wanted to hide. I had never really been ill before, although three years before I had a kidney removed due to an unknown childhood condition that meant it didn't grow properly – I kind of felt like I did when waking up from that operation. Dazed and confused.

I'm not sure if I told anyone, if I did, nothing happened. The next day I felt a bit better and the day after that I was back to normal. It was a very powerful experience.

We landed at Ben Gurion Airport in Tel Aviv fairly late at night. We were met by a cool-looking guy called Uri and a beautiful female, whose name I forget. They were very chilled and happy. There were maybe eight of us or so on the flight from London, we had exited the plane to a heat I mistook for that from the jet engines. It was still hot and humid as I climbed aboard their little bus, we had a two-hour journey to our Kibbutz north of Kiryat Shmona, near Mount Hermon. Much nearer Damascus or Beirut than Tel Aviv.

Only twenty minutes into the journey, we stopped – to pick up Soldiers, with big black rifles slung on their shoulders. One got in, sat next to me, plonked his gun down, pointing up and resting on my leg.

I was literally staring down the barrel, it was a Colt M16 (A2) assault rifle, an improved version of the M16's used in Vietnam -apparently. We picked up several on the way, it was customary, in fact, it was expected of you, IDF military were everywhere and if they pointed to the road (in England, we stuck out a thumb), you were obliged to give them a lift. Of course, due to their conscription, just about anyone over eighteen had spells in fatigues. I was spellbound by the girls, all tooled up in military green, a fantasy I never knew I had.

We arrived in pitch black in an area that looked and felt like Dartmoor in Devon, and it had cooled dramatically. A prison with palm trees. Lots of security checks before we were allowed in. Someone mentioned they had a rocket come over from Lebanon a few nights back. We were also reminded how we were not allowed out when dark for fear of not seeing the red triangles that marked out the minefields.

The next day after a lovely breakfast in the canteen we were given a talk and allocated our jobs, Matt was given Kitchen duties, a 6 am start – LOL! I was allocated avocado picking, 4 am – FOUR!!! Four??? Oh, so my nights at the makeshift disco in a bomb shelter were to be ruined by having to turn in earlier than others, obviously missing out on all the action.

There are many stories I could talk of, but they would deviate too far from the purpose of the book.

Having said that, and bearing in mind my mate was a bomber...

We went scorpion hunting in the Golan Heights, it was too irresistible, they were to be found under rocks, so nothing seemed more of a better idea than slipping your fingers under the rocks to find out if you were lucky. It would have been a typical idea of Matts but, actually, it was mine.

We did find some, little golden ones, I wanted the big black ones, we had some miniature bottles and thought our new friends in the kibbutz would want to see them. Turns out, the big black ones were relatively harmless but the small golden ones not.

That aside, we were surrounded by the leftovers of war, burnt-out tanks, field guns, and ammunition, loads of it, live rounds, belts of shiny brass shells clipped together with the lead-coloured bullets protruding. We also found lots of black cylindrical grainy pellets that turned out to be Cordite – explosives. Matt was ecstatic. Obviously, we agreed it was a good idea to bring them back to our shared bedroom hut.

Someone showed us how we could have fun with the bullets. What you do is get two pairs of pliers, grab the shell with one and the bullet with the other, wiggle the bullet so it becomes loose, and pull it out careful not to spill the gunpowder within.

Carefully place a few shells, open end up, near a sleeping friend, light some matches and drop them in each one. They will fizz through the gunpowder with a nice soporific hum until they reach the primer. Then, holy crap!!! Live, loud, terrifying gunfire all around, right here, right now - Bang, Bang, Bang. How our sleeping friends laughed.

Then things got serious, Matt had found a large Nescafe tin, bucket size with a snap-on lid, and he had a plan. "Mate, if we ram this with the cordite pellets and pierce a hole in the lid, light one, chuck it in, and whack the lid on, it will be epic." We were both nineteen and stupid – but happy. We knew of a bomb shelter away from the living areas, seemingly uncared for, lots of weeds around it unlike the others, but always unlocked and free to enter. Ideal.

So, after placing it deep down a dark corridor, we did as Matt suggested, half-filled the coffee tin with cordite pellets, lit one, threw it in, and rammed the pierced lid on top. We ran back and ducked into the nearest corner we could poke our heads round to watch the experiment play out.

It was like an inverted Apollo mission, getting ready for lift-off. First a six-inch Bunsen burner on turbo, a loud hiss, then a two-foot burst of jet engine, then one hell of a boom, the lid flew into the ceiling, the tin split open like an accelerated flower and yellow/white projectiles shot out everywhere. Then came the shimmer, we laughed with nervousness, the shimmer advanced quickly and smacked into our faces. Instant burn.

Alarms went off around the whole camp, we ran out of the bunker and noticed smoke billowing out of some air vents. Boy were we in trouble.

Still, they won't have a clue who did it. We will keep quiet – and maybe not do it again. We casually entered the disco for a couple or three swift glugs on the Arak. Didn't get that far, people were pointing and laughing, we hadn't even noticed each other. Bright red, we were both bright red in the faces like we had a severe peanut reaction. Shit, we were so in trouble.

Yes, we were. Threats of deportation and prosecution but, surprisingly, we weren't the first, and Uri, our guy, seemed to find our stupid faces funny. We had a disco ban for a week, that was it.

Back to something relevant.

It was about six months in, we were loving life and visiting the most amazing places. The Dead Sea, Masada, The Red Sea, Jerusalem, Bethlehem, and Jericho. We will take a very quick drive through Jericho, the oldest city in the world, they said. It can get a bit rough in the West Bank, so just a quick one. As I said before, we were only 19 and had absolutely no idea of the Israeli / Palestinian situation, certainly didn't have any affiliation of support with either side, and still don't. As we were driving through Jericho, one of our guides shouted, 'No, not good - go back' to the driver. A gang of kids had appeared, they didn't seem angry, they were laughing happily in fact, but they were hurling rocks and stones at us, some had catapults. We three-point turned in haste to the sound of clunk, bosh, ping as we were getting hit - no windows were smashed, nobody hurt but we were all happy to head somewhere else. Good to say I've been to Jericho, better to say I've been stoned in Jericho especially when conversation dries up at dinner parties.

One month later, or so, I woke up in a fuzz, like a blur, like in some kind of psychedelic lava lamp. Everything was going slow, my voice echoed again, I was as weak as hell. I felt down, very down, and anxious. I didn't go to work, I didn't get up – couldn't get up, 'shit, what is wrong with me?'

I didn't get better, this went on for a week, I was seen by the doctor, they took bloods. I was dying. This was so bad; I was obviously dying. They didn't know what was wrong, but I saw a note that the Kibbutz doctor had written, Kidney failure it said. Oh man, I am dying. The doctor told me she didn't know what it was, but I needed to go to a hospital quickly, in Haifa. They called an ambulance, and I was bundled in, feeling awful – exactly like I felt the day after those injections.

On the way to the hospital, we passed the red triangle markers, I knew this as there was only the one road going West. Selfishly, I remember hoping we would lose control on a corner, roll into a minefield and we would all blow up – instant, not a gradual descent to death in some foreign hospital.

I was kept in hospital for a few days before they advised I go back to the UK, they couldn't find anything wrong, my Kidney was ok. So, I did, still feeling incredibly weak and fuzzy, dazed, and confused, I flew back, alone.

Around two weeks later, my doctor informed me it was Yuppie Flu. Yuppie Flu! What, 'it's all in my head?' 'Fuck off with that bollocks'. 'No way'. This was something very powerful and real. Oh yes, he said, Chronic Fatigue Syndrome, Myalgic Encephalomyelitis, Post Viral Syndrome, one of those anyway. They are syndromes, conditions we can't really test for, a lot of teenagers are getting it, you tick all the boxes, but you should be ok after a year or so – you may want to try hypnotherapy, he said.

It lasted a good three years and I still get some of the symptoms if I pick up a cold or flu, weird, trippy. That's my 'Long Covid' experience. More likely 'Long Vax'.

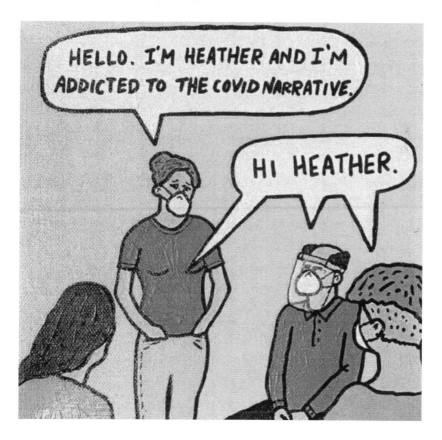

11. The Spotty Little Hitler Phenomenon

Give someone a hat of authority, or an armband, even better. Not just anyone, try those with Short Person Syndrome, the Napoleon Complex. In the UK we have a particular type of 'copper', far removed from the gentle giants we had, the Bobbies, your man on the street corner looking after us protecting us, assisting the elderly with directions, clipping the urchin around the ear for nicking a jam doughnut. No, we have - or increasingly *had*, due to the recent emergence of the baseball-capped, baton-wielding Robocops - a breed of either 4ft, fat females, resembling R2D2, or 6'6" skinny beanpole spotty males with the top of their trousers all pleated due to the over fastened belt, with self-made holes, tightened around a non-existent waist keeping the ill-fitting waistband in place – like a curtain pole. Too much visible sock. Them.

They were trained to stand in groups, and all had to stick their thumbs into the front of the armholes of their flak jackets – imagine a sooty Dick Van Dyke frog-legging his way over the roofs going all 'chim, chimminy, churoo guvnor'. I guess they were taught this to stop them just randomly hitting out with a reflexive jerk as they spoke at you. They were so rude and aggressive, full of attitude, and domineering behaviour without any physical domination. They would have had a lifetime of inferiority fuelled by the bullies at school, insults, and laughed at – this is their revenge. Personally, I detected they also felt stupid at times, vulnerable (as they should), I thought the thumbs in flak jackets were also a little reassuring self-cuddle. I was always tempted to just push them over and watch them desperately trying to unhook their flexed thumbs in time to prevent the inevitable concrete-to-spotty chin collision.

So, it seemed the best way for a tyrannical regime to control the people was to use the people most charged with pent-up anger and aggression, ready to take revenge on the world like the perfect psychopath. Brainwash them with more victimhood and noble causes for the greater good that will make them heroes, legends in their own lunchtime, and you have powerful law enforcement – after all, what protester would punch a fat lady dwarf?

This tactic applies to Antifa, BLM, Trans-Rights, MyBodyMyChoice etc, always the same whipped up over excited and unintelligent victims, give them some flags, press the button, and watch them go mental. They will kill for their cause, ask them about their cause and they can't explain it.

Back to the hats and armbands, or the florescent jackets as donned by The Covid Marshals.

Trained in unarmed combat, tactical field operators, skilled in the arts of control and restraint, fonts of knowledge with anything Covid, can spot a virus, isolate it, and go in for the kill, fearlessly and swift. The A team, big, strong, and reassuring. Marshals empowered to direct the people scattering in fear, they make the decisions, they keep order, they keep you safe. I don't know how you work your way up to Marshal level but can imagine you are the cream of the forces, topflight SAS types.

Hmmm, the ones we had were either poor students, middle-aged ladies, or friendless 'XBoxer' men (not men who used to box but men who think they are invincible digital warriors slaying dragons) fresh from their smelly bedrooms at their Mum's house.

Somehow, these people were allowed to wear the jackets of the Marshals. Bless the students and the ladies, really, their hearts were in the right place naively. They knew nothing about Covid but if you asked why they were asking you to stand five paces to the right or to keep moving along the path, they would say 'Coz Covid', they were good at it. 'Coz Covid' with a smile and a frown worked well in most cases. 'Coz Covid' disarmed people quite easily, it was a conversation stopper, people just couldn't top it, it was like saying 'End Of', after announcing your stupid opinion. Nothing is allowed to come back 'Coz, End Of'.

It became a daily pastime, quite fun. I would go looking for them, it was always the same 6-8, always in pairs. My 'faves' were the smelly bedroom boys. They all wore glasses and strange facial hair arrangements. They hated me, as I would stop them and initially ask for help, they, being the experts, such as 'Excuse me Field Marshal, can you tell me why the RT-PCR differs from Mullis's original?' or maybe a light discussion – 'what parallels do you see with your job and the Stasi of post-war East Germany?' – I could tell they would compete as to who was the most assertive, who had the best quip and who could put me in my place. If stuttered, they instantly lost. They often stuttered. Initially, they seemed keen to help, but then probably around encounter three, I would see them approaching me and mysteriously veer from their path, like they had some kind of incoming missile warning system.

I would sometimes give chase, talking to the back of their numbskull heads but they had obviously hatched a plan to disengage, or their bosses had prescribed it during their debriefing sessions.

One day to my surprise they were walking towards me and on sighting their nemesis, they sped up, sticking to a direct path my way, they had a jolly spring in their step, confident smiles, eyes like Tom out of Tom and Jerry with an evil intent. As they drew near up came the fumbling hands to their chest, 'Where is it, where is the fucking thing, I mustn't look down to locate it, come on, in training I got it first time'. I think one did it first time, but the other clumsy fool had to look down after twice grabbing his lanyard. They were tooling up. They were bloody armed! Right in the middle of their chests were Body Cams, they came right up to me with red lights flashing. I was bemused at the fat one obviously filming some clouds above due to his sub-sternal tilt. I am sure they have a video montage of me sitting on a server somewhere.

Britain's army of clampdown officers with their 'up until then' inferiority complex was not always confined to uniform. Anyone with any authority over their space would become superhuman, having been given their moral superiority. Café owners, bar staff, bus drivers, bouncers, and people in their pathetic little bubbles. 'Oi, you – mask up now or you're barred. Move away now!' You could sense them reaching for their officially issued Tazer.

The thing is, if these people gladly developed their higher standing over you, they would be the neighbours informing the authorities about you – the informers, the collaborators, the traitors.

Maybe time to check if Amazon stocks 'Tar and Feather' kits.

12. Mask Wars

I knew we were in trouble when I saw the first Mask/Handbag leopard skin matching combo, proudly worn by a school mother. The Stockholm Syndrome victims were starting to love their shackles.

I was warning people they were likely to encourage a lovely little bacterial respiratory infection with their grubby over-fiddled face pads. 'It's better than getting 'Covid'', they would say, not realising the irony of it probably being the same thing. It was too late though; the latest craze had hit town -everyone was doing it. C'mon baby, do the locomotion. I thought Bonce-Boppers were better.

Yes, I did it for about two weeks, leading up to my Supermarket 'recce', I very quickly realised what it was all about. How do the architects of this attack on us really know the levels of compliance? Well, they just count how many sheep walk around with their farmer's stamp. How badly are people falling for this? How many are like me and my Parler friends? Just look outside, what percentage are covering their faces in turquoise paper? I would say 99%. The government and their 'SAGE' nudge units must have been high-fiving like beach volleyball players. Their plan was working like a dream – Ha, Suckers! It was 'normal'.

'The hell it's normal', I thought, as did another. 'Let's fight this bollocks'. We set up, on the new Telegram platform, 'The Smile High Club'. The idea was simple, we would gather as many as possible to descend on a pre-chosen Supermarket at a given date and time range, as individuals, not a protest, not a pack, not to look organised. We would be bare-faced, hence the smile.

We would all enter individually between, say 10 am and 10:30 and do some shopping, not much maybe a couple of items but we would all ensure that at least one of us was in every isle. We had to remind people what NORMAL looks like, you can't let that slip permanently. Often, we would have 20-30 people in one store, generally, we managed to get in with minimal confrontation, but you could see the increasingly raised eyebrows of the security staff — well, that's all you could see anyway - and some fear in their eyes. 'Holy Shit, what's happening, why on my shift?'

We would coordinate each target with military precision over several weeks. Then the numbers dropped, the novelty was wearing off. People started to have other things to do. They would request different days or times to suit their needs. 'This is a war, people' 'It aint much but it's having an effect' 'Come on, keep it up'. It was having an effect, we would speak to people in the shops, especially the ones with their noses poking free. There were lots of those - 'mask-cheats'. 'I'm wearing my mask, but not, I'm complying, but not, I'm rebreathing my CO_2, but not'.

The 'semi-masked' were the easiest. 'Go on, take it off', I would say with a visible smile. They would look back, intrigued, and carry on. I would pass them again. 'Take it off man, you know you want to' - often they did. Whether that provoked a path to awakening I don't know, but it gave some people that little jolt of confidence they needed, that permission. They can say 'no'.

It was working yet the Smile High Club was falling apart. 'I can't do Tuesday at six as we tend to have dinner then', 'I have children and they need their routine'. I think I killed the project by publicly barking back 'Do you think the fucking French Resistance had this?? Do you think they had requests from British Command saying they were 'coming in at 03 hundred hours, prepare a landing strip, coordinates: 50°57'7" N 1°51.381' E, ground cover required' and they replied 'Ah, sorry, erm, a tad inconvenient, we tend to be sleeping at that time, could you make it 09:30, after breakfast perhaps?'

The Smile high Club disbanded. He Who Dares Whines.

The daily confrontation with the underequipped security staff would go something like this... ..' Sorry, you can't come in without a mask'. "I don't wear masks." 'Are you exempt'. "Probably." 'What does that mean'. "I guess it means that my body breathes IN Oxygen and OUT Carbon Dioxide, I am not a tree." 'So, are you exempt?'. "From what?." 'Wearing a Mask'. "I expect so, I think my doctor recommends O2, excuse me, time is tight, I need to do my shopping." 'You can't come in without a mask'. "Why?." 'It's mandatory here – unless you are exempt'. "Of course, I'm exempt, and it's not the law then is it?"... ... at this point, you would just walk past them, invariably to 'tuts' and 'mutterings' from other customers, often worse. I would often film these encounters for entertainment but soon grew tired and cross, so just ended up barging past with a loud 'NOPE, WON'T' before they could speak.

If one didn't have the time for such fun, you could 'play the game' and flash an exemption picture on your phone downloaded from official government websites – nothing was required to prove exemption, you just self-declare, mainly because we weren't trees. They had some flowery lanyards for 'the exempt' but they tended to be used by the 'disabled', people felt sorry for them, 'bless them, they can't be protected, yet they must be so vulnerable, such a shame'. On that subject, though, and what was more sinister was the overprotective masking of 'people in care', you would see them on outings barely breathing, and then there were those masking their children. 'That is Child Abuse', we found ourselves telling parents, 'Shame on You' – probably a tad unfair as these people were brainwashed and terrified.

There were a lot of 'little Hitlers', over-excited security staff, we would target them for fun. Especially the smart-arse doorman at LEGO, he was supercharged, you could really wind him up, make him call for backup that never came – due to the frequency of requests. I also knew of a tactic that my female friend used which was pretty insensitive in normal times, but we were (are) in a war, sometimes you fight bullshit with bullshit. 'Hello, hello, Oi, You! Lady! Stop! Why are you not wearing your mask?' 'I was brutally raped as a student, he put his hand over my face, over my mouth and nose, I couldn't breathe as I tried to scream, It destroyed me, but, if you insist....'. They didn't insist.

This really wasn't just at home, we managed to grab a flight to Portugal for a long weekend before the looming travel restrictions. They were Maskaholics there, loved 'em, full-on virtue signalling, super proud bearers. I made the mistake upon landing, in the nearest supermarket of trying to breathe. Something within thought it necessary. I had barely popped my nose out for a couple of seconds and bash – confrontation, a shouty Portuguese 'house frau', in English, she knew, 'You think you are special, you selfish pig, you come here to infect us and don't give a sheet'. Not sure what kind of sheet she wanted me to give, and to whom, but gathered she was pretty cross so dumped my shopping, bar the vinho, and made for the 'five items or less' exit. We didn't venture out much, they were just annoyingly acquiescent – obviously better than us.

The designs were proving popular and yet divisive, my wife and I would have great debates on what was best to show one's defiance when in a hospital setting where your concern over a loved one overrode the need to fight. We both had very close relatives who were quite ill – nothing to do with viruses. I would stick to the turquoise paper one, incorrectly worn, but worn. She thought the full-face curved Perspex window variety, with a headband saying 'Covid Mask' on it (?) more rebellious as she could show her face. Personally, I preferred to hide my shame.

There were the snoods for people who said they don't wear masks and the ones with the side vent and filter – for those thinking they were in the SAS, then there were the double cylinder filter respirator types for those thinking they were in Chornobyl. There were some who double-upped, a few who triple-upped, some thought it great to have ones with funny mouths, or skeleton jaws. Others liked to ensure they were colour-coordinated.

All of the above were waiting outside the school gates every day, collaborators, sheep. They really annoyed me and obviously, my selfishness really annoyed them.

Sitting at a restaurant or pub was always fine as the airborne viral droplets cruised at a cool 5'2" altitude and above. Should you need to stand, obviously masking up kept you – and more importantly, others safe. I remember one hero entering an open-fronted restaurant. His table was just one or two steps inside. We were sitting one table further in. We saw him happy and committed to the move, he was already leaning towards the table in an unstoppable phase of movement -the laws of physics had kicked in. The happy face turned to horror as he realised that he was unmasked and a step inside was imminent, he was well in the viral level and about to commit manslaughter. With one finger, he managed to hook up his t-shirt neck, hoist it upright and over his nose. Momentum took him to the safety of his seat, his eyes relaxed into relief, he had made it, a cool finger flick release of the virus defying clothing – to a round of deserved applause.

Masks were also great for the adolescents who had been indoctrinated into victims, with victimhood, they had anxiety. For anxiety, hiding behind your mask works well, you can venture outside. You can gather amongst others and 'be kind' together (with hate).

Antifa and every other 'controlled opposition' such as 'The Patriot Front' in the US and 'Just Stop Oil' in the UK are big fans of masks – they can do their thing whilst hiding the fact they are sons of prominent Democrats or the daughters of Hollywood celebs, they are generally from a well to do background. I am bamboozled as to how the deep state players think Patriots would wear masks – of course they don't, but then equally bamboozled how their fake MAGA far-right militias also wear Fed Beige Chinos. Come on boys, try harder.

13. SUBSTACKS 1-7

2021/2022/2023, three years of battle, verbal battle, written battle, mainly on WhatsApp. I really tried. As much as I tried, I failed. I am really talking about my brother and my son (he with his own family) – I really tried to wake them into some kind of action. I may have had more success with my dad, but his dementia was really kicking in. Brother took the piss and argued about everything, and my son just ignored everything, however, he says he didn't take a jab – the only one from my side of my family.

The result, for me was an overriding frustration, discombobulation, a constant obsessive disbelief at their nonchalance – it hurt physically and emotionally. My brain was going to explode. It needed a pressure valve. I noticed something called 'Substack', a self-publishing platform for articles, I had read a few, not really knowing they were Substacks. I realised the beauty of the concept when I finally looked into it, so I thought I would try it out. I just started writing about what was occupying my amygdala, the almond shaped processing centre for my anxieties (part of my limbic system in my brain) - just because it was easier. It just flows out.

I found it cathartic and cheaper than paying a counsellor, or psychiatrist. Actually, I did try private counselling, but the counsellors were never on my page, I had to explain why I was in such a state, why I was so stressed, and that meant opening pandora's box. 'It must be difficult for you to hold such views', they would say – they would think 'hmm, delusional, paranoid, fruitcake'.

Yes, Substack allowed me some catharsis. I was offloading to an imaginary listener, and it helped – a lot.

I wrote seven 'newsletters' as they were referred to, sometimes completely veering away from my family struggles, sometimes my 'hopium' got out of control, and often the grammar could be better, but I think they encapsulated a crazy clown world that we all resided in. (and still do).

This is Chaz667's Newsletter, a newsletter called –

WTF! Wake up, your house in on fire!!!

You must feel like this some days. I find myself completely alone yet surrounded by what look like normal people doing their normal things in their normal lives - as if everything was normal. Actually, I know some of these people. Some are family, they keep sending me pictures of their happy carefree lives.

Yet, their house is on fire! I have tried to tell them, their house in on fire and they are in grave danger. They don't seem to give a damn.

Have I got mad? Nope, their neighbours house is also ablaze, and I can see the casualties. Can they not see what I see? Can they not even see the smoke or smell some smouldering BS?

If they can't, that must be due to some disability - surely. I guess inability, the lack of ability to look sideways from everything mainstream feeding their narrow 'input funnels'. So, they are shielded from everything telling them their house is on fire. Total insulation and I just can't penetrate it.

So, maybe they can smell but just won't see. Maybe they decide to ignore the strong pungent smell of burning - why would they do that?

Is it a fear that they may just see something too hellish to deal with, maybe their social circle or work colleagues have some kind of a death wish pact that will cast them out like leapers should they break out and sound a small alarm? Oh, the shame!

What if they know their house is on fire and their children are in danger, yet somehow they still won't take action??

How about, in my normal world, I tell them "I know some people who have planned to harm your children, and your friends' children, I can show you where to see who those people are and how they are going to do it." In my world and maybe the world 3 years ago they would say "oh my god, who? where? what? - show me now !!"

But they are not, they don't want to know.

Is this a gene deletion issue, a cognitive dissonance, a manipulated fear, a clever brainwashing psychological operation, something in the water - or all the above?

There are some of us who somehow missed all of that, how was that?

Like many of you, I am dreading the next meet up with these people. The ones who want you to shut up and just be normal. For me, it's happening next week, and I feel like I'm going to go absolutely mental with them - fall out with them all and then just sound like a crazy purple wearing hocus pocus flat earther.

Let's see.

Bro, wake up and do something, your house is on fire.

Some background... and a cunning plan

CHAZ667

2 AUG 2022

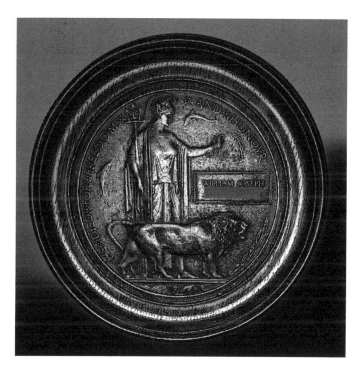

This hangs on my bedroom wall, I never really thought much about it until recently, and actually reading what it says. My great grandfather, shot by a sniper in WW 1.

More about this later, but I think I should briefly give some background into my writings. I guess this is intended to be mainly cathartic, partly to record an aspect of this most amazing, yet mind-blowing, time in history and maybe to resonate with many others going through these very bizarre experiences. Maybe this will help because, God knows, there is no manual for what we are going through. It's not as if someone out there has previously experienced a full-on information war between covert patriots and an evil, media owning, cabal and worked out how to navigate through it, undoing cognitive dissonances at will, and leaving us a handy step by step 'idiots guide'.

I am also going mad with the stubbornness, ignorance and naivety of my brother who refuses to wake up and do something to protect his children's future. To a lesser but equally frustratingly my son who has his own young children.

I have been at it for over 2 years now and there are 2 reasons why I should give up:

1. My relationship with them is in real jeopardy and people close to me tell me to just give up antagonising them.
2. I believe the White Hats are in control, so it doesn't really matter in the great scheme of things.

However, there are at least 3 reasons why not to give up:

1. We used to love watching the 'footy' together and talk about sport and drink beer- they are missing out on the biggest most complex end to end 'sporting' battle in human history, and I would love to enjoy it with them. But nope, I can't really even discuss it without them shutting down - and it's so bloody exciting, I just want to share the experience.
2. We now know how pre-WW2 Germany happened without everyone laughing and ignoring all that Nazi nonsense and

instead falling for a massive psyop machine. There is that analogy, you know, about ever thinking what you would have done if you were around then, or during apartheid, and that it would be exactly whatever you are doing right now. I actually want to prevent them having to answer to their children in a few years' time - 'but how come you didn't know what was happening, it must have been obvious' or 'what did you do to fight against it?'.

3. To actually help them do the most basic digital warrior stuff if they can't take direct action, it is necessary. Although I believe in Devolution and Q and the plan, and see it playing out daily, I still know more people need to reach that point of awakening for it all to happen smoothly (as if something like this can go smoothly).

There are other reasons, such as stopping them getting injected again with the latest booster or Monkeypox / Marburg jab, wearing useless masks, joining in with their friend's virtue signalling etc. Also, to stop my personal anguish and pain having to watch them with their heads firmly deep in the sand while getting on with their happy care free lives - that people like us have strived to protect for over 2 bloody years, suffering the abuse and hate that goes with it.

So, not giving up wins.

I knew about a month into the 'pandemic' that it was staged. I then became aware very quickly that PCR was fraudulent. Prior to that I watched Trump getting cheated out of an election and could see tyranny was on its way. Once I got a few more facts together,

I thought, naturally, to warn my family and stop them from taking the death jabs. So rather than our usual beer and facetime footy chat, I thought I would tell them I needed to tell them something very important and it would take a while. I had a long pre-prepared script (how can you explain the whole deep state agenda and the counter plan, off the cuff, nowadays it would take about a month, non-stop!).

So, my brother called it a 'lecture' and has taken the piss ever since. My Son listened and seemed to take it in while his eyes were saying 'shit, my dad's gone mental'. I tried to get them on Parler, and then Telegram after the DS took down the former - even that didn't raise suspicions. Brother called me 'Telegram Sam' with lots of hilarious 'crying with laughter' emojis. The message was always, don't listen to me, here, go find out yourself. But they don't.

So, this has gone on for two years and there have been many times when we have obviously fallen out, ignoring each other. My brother got himself jabbed twice with AZ, thinking the Chimpanzee adenovirus was better than the baby foetal cells. Oh how he laughed when he told me he wasn't yet swinging through the trees (please get Monkeypox, pleeeeeese - don't mean that - I do). His wife got 'team Pfizers'. They would mask the kids but not get them jabbed. Son says he has not taken a shot, but he was a very keen mask wearer, his wife has. I have worn myself out sending info by email, phone or WhatsApp and it is now obvious they have hatched a behaviour modification plan to ignore me if I say anything conspiratorial and reward with great encouragement anything about footy. I also get bombarded with lots of pics of happy smiley families enjoying their fantastic lives.

Then Matt LeTissier, a footballer, suddenly announced there was something nefarious going on with the virus, the tests, and the lockdowns, he felt we were being lied to!! He was right, of course. Within hours my brother decided it was indeed true, we had been lied to, they had staged a pandemic, the BBC and our politicians maybe don't love us all!!

He apologised and I thought, great, now we can talk and get through this together, enjoy ups and downs and watch the White Hats stunning plan play out -leading up to the big scare event before the storm and then the glorious biblical finale. Err, no, he gets they lied about Covid but everything else is just me getting carried away with my new freedom fighter friends' crazy ideas - surely if anything like that was true it would be on the telly, he would obviously think. Since then, it's been, why don't you just get on with your life like us, you're missing out! It would be right to assume I have been very active over the last two years.

So, I have informed and warned about issues at the Borders, Cashless societies, Vax Passports, Russia being the good guys, Ukraine the baddies, Biolabs, Texas shootings and other false flags, WEF, WHO, UN, Hunter and the other Bidens, Clintons, BLM, Antifa, Soros - EVERYTHING and there is zero interest, often nonsensical arguments fired back. Also, I have excitedly enthused about Q, Devolution, WH operations, Infiltrations, Musk, the Alliance, the storm that is coming - NOTHING, just a look in reaction that could be equal to me explaining that I have a drainage problem in the kitchen, no real questions... I really do wonder about this gene deletion thing, where is the critical thinking? Where is the curiosity?

Anyway, we are due to visit them all in 4 days for a big birthday celebration - how is this going to go without me chucking in a load of truth bombs - and being the mad villain? It's a big worry.

So, my cunning plan.

The plaque above is something given to me by my equally blinkered Mother. I have had it for years without it really having any impact on me. Until now. This is our great and great great grandfather who gave up his life for our freedom. It says so - 'He died for Freedom'. When you hold it and feel the bronze it has an effect. It is meant as a warning to us that our freedoms can be taken away unless we are prepared to die fighting for it. It is already in progress though, our governments are not working for us now, they work for the World Economic Forum, and they are going to Build Back Better (for them).

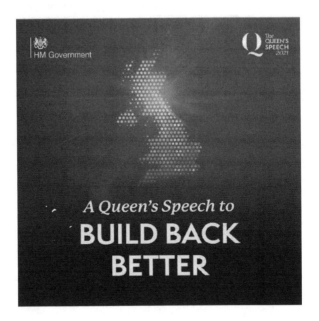

My cunning plan is really a cheesy guilt trip attempt, let them hold it and read it and reflect. He died for us, maybe they can just wake up and do something to protect their children's' future. Maybe they will start to look for the truth and then realise their house is on fire. Maybe.

Will let you know how I get on...

Substack 3

I've just returned, 5 hours without aircon on an English motorway in 35 degrees. It's summer, just summer, not a climate crisis - but it was bloody hot. Luckily, I live by the sea.

We all met at my parents' house last week for my mother's 80th birthday and I have been anxious about it for a long time, mainly due to my pent up anger that they have refused to join any dots and wake up. Mother and brother both jabbed. Brother knows they staged a pandemic, woke for a bit, then fell asleep again. My cunning plan was to shame them with the 'dying for freedom' plaque awarded to my mother's grandfather.

I just can't help it, anything anybody mentions about 'life' and I make a comment steering attention towards the evil globalists and/or the ignorant masses. I think I did it within 5 minutes of meeting my brother for the first time since Jan 2020 (our last big reunion which was a barrel of laughs and carefree boozing). This time, we were watching football and they 'took the knee' before the first half. At the start of the second half, I wondered out loud which pose they may adopt before kicking off, I guessed the 'tree pose'. I didn't happen but it kicked off some sibling beef. Him saying 'I was looking forward to being with you but not if you're going to cause arguments', so we had a frosty 20 mins before all going to the beach.

We both swam in the sea and messed around like we used to (before they attacked us). I started to relax and enjoy it and felt the need for a truce. Then he asked me what I thought will happen with Russia, Ukraine, China, Taiwan etc etc. So off I go again, explaining the whole Deep State agenda and my belief in a White Hat sting, then I went on to moralise about our personal responsibilities and duties, mentioning our great granddad, suggesting our children in the future will ask why we didn't know or act... .Then I brought up a recent interaction that made me laugh with face planting frustration. I had warned my brother, and also my son, about the 'drag queen story time' (can't bring myself to capitalise them) events, touring the US and UK, and the sexualisation of our young children - the grooming. I hoped that by bringing the children into the equation, they may actually take some counter action and fight back. Instead, after several prompts for a reaction, I got this response - enjoy.

Peter Pan was always a woman in tiny shorts

Widow Twankey was always a man - we were taken to pantomime at 5

How about don't take your kids to the library if you're worried.

I've asked my kids if they are being encouraged to become a drag queen in PSHE. And no, they are not.

It rendered me speechless for a couple of days. Anyway, between waves, I reinforced that this thing runs much deeper and is far more sinister AND it's not about YOUR kids who may have missed such delights, it's about ALL kids FFS!

Something clicked, we got on well for the two days before they left for home - I didn't get the chance to get the plaque out but he initiated further conversation a few times and something felt different.

The day after he returned, he actually sent me something from Telegram and it was about the C-19 virus and the Jabs being bioweapons! - a very good interview with Dr Richard Fleming (https://rumble.com/v1f9xll-dr.-richard-fleming-exposes-the-vaccine-and-covid-bioweapons.html).

This was a great surprise and, for me, a significant turnaround.

But here is the biggest surprise. I didn't know how much I needed my mother to believe in me. Always the black sheep, always the one causing problems, and seemingly, the one not making the most of my qualifications - and for the last two and a half years, the one upsetting the neighbours and friends with my selfish refusal to wear masks, take PCR tests and crazy ideas about governments wanting to kill us with death jabs.

I didn't know this until I suggested she watched the same Dr Fleming interview. It is very 'evidenced science' based and objective - you just can't argue against it - but, at over an hour long, I doubted she would get beyond 5 minutes. She sat alone in a back room watching on my phone (please God, nobody call me, not right now!), I could hear it playing at a distance and could see her concentrating hard- when peeking.

I was upstairs when I heard her enter the kitchen where my youngest daughter was. All I could hear was her saying "Wow, wow,

wow, my god, I've been brainwashed, we've all been brainwashed." She had tears in her eyes and was visibly stunned. I have tried for two and a half years to get her to accept this. She suddenly knew what I - and my wife - had gone through for so long, she suddenly knew how we had been ridiculed and hated. She suddenly knew we were right all along.

I told her that we have probably saved hundreds of kids from taking these jabs, poster-ing around schools at 2AM, leafleting directly, writing to headmasters, meeting headmasters, writing to parents, entering jab centres, closing jabbing events, standing at roundabouts with yellow boards, organising mask-less shopping etc and just getting abuse, hate and ridicule back.

Then it happened, out of the blue and for the first time in about four decades, I just lost it in floods of tears, a massive release of emotion (I just don't get emotional), she became apologetic and put her arms around me acknowledging my (our) suffering and effort. I didn't know it, but I needed this so much. My daughter watched in polite confusion but also with a strange nonchalance.

When things calmed, she spoke of her friends and how she could not possibly even try to tell them - "yes, no, don't try, it's a bloody nightmare!" She also said she has had no idea what to tell them what I do, workwise (will explain at a later date but basically, it's this!). All her friends are always so proud of what their offspring have achieved - I couldn't think also - hate the word Truther, thought about Researcher, toyed with Investigator, but I now know what I should tell her - I work with US Military Intelligence!!

Substack 4

Even if the truth was a wet fish slapping the face of a 'Normie', they can't and won't believe it exists. Not at first anyway, and not even after a few more slaps. Something deep and visceral needs to be hit hard. It seems to me that people have their own deep-seated switch and everyone's different. If we are to wake people into action, sometimes the house being on fire isn't enough. Take my brother, he suddenly woke, with an apology to me, after 18 months of me shouting because a footballer also told him his house was on fire. This says something more about sibling rivalry and a perceived acquiescence that caused his unwillingness to listen, but a footballer who he looked up to..... well now it makes sense to listen and hear the actual message! Bingo.

What I have found is that you may think the eagle has landed with a big 'aha experience' that leads to a complete switch in behaviour - action and urgency to deal with the fire maybe. But, even knowing that PCR was a fraud, the virus was pretty benign and the coerced injections incredibly nefarious, eventually they slump back into pre-awakening mode. The deeply ingrained 'knowledge' that our government loves us, and the BBC won't lie to us. Everything is just fine and dandy. Hear no evil, see no evil...

Having said that, there is a real change with my brother, at the moment, he seems interested in my perspective and in my world - which is currently being a full-time digital soldier in a world-wide battle between good and evil- epic fantasy end of civilization movie stuff, but real! We are almost at the precipice, and it is nail biting as hell. But he is contributing. I am pretty sure that his internal trigger had switched when I suggested his children, a few years from now, will be asking him what he did in our version of pre-war Nazi Germany, how could he not have known??? This really seems to have worked.

I am starting to have successful red-pilling experiences that were not planned, so there are people out there who really know nothing, but they do have that feeling something is not right. If you get one of those at the right time - it is easy and very rewarding - I will detail both experiences in the next episode but, as a heads up, one was my nice neighbour flying stripy flags for the 'opposition' at a protest for a local drag queen story hour (child grooming event). The other is a CBT therapist trying to fix my 'social anxiety'. Both flipped without me trying. Both experiences need fully explaining so that's to come next time.

You may have read Episode 3, where I had an amazing experience watching my mother suddenly realise that she has been brainwashed by the government - and my subsequent emotional event.

We just connected again today and spoke about the brilliant video she watched that turned her world upside down - her great and beautiful awakening. We spoke about the absurdity of the fantastic new booster coming soon to save us in the UK. The dual strain booster, you know, the one that does both Covid and Omicron!! We then agreed that it was another massive con, a bioweapon that targets Omicron BA1 - the first Omicron strain - the strain that is now ancient history, we have had its grandchildren (BA 2.5) come and go since then and it's great grandchildren (BA 4) and now it's great great grandchild (BA god knows what) - so it was awesome to agree what a load of bollocks they are trying to sell us.

Then she says - of course we will take it though as we are

VULNERABLE!

FFS

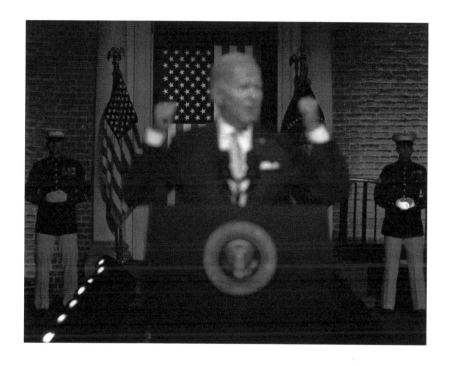

Substack 5

About 25 years ago I paid a lot of money to see the world's biggest supergroup play at Wembley stadium. To watch the fantastic anti-war and anti-fascist visuals behind these mega rock stars was an education in how to red-pill the masses before red-pilling existed, it was the wake-the-fuck up message behind the music. The red and black fascist tones of a dark and sinister dictator in their film flickered behind the drummer, with marching jackboots, pounding oppression to the beat. As a punk 10 years before, I learnt about Nazism, Racism, Communism, Royalty, even

Nicaraguan revolutions, etc etc - Rock stars did what they always did going back to Dylan, this is where we learnt about the truth, this is why 'we don't need no education' - it's indoctrination by oppressors isn't it, and we only really find out when we listen to the lyrics from people brave enough to speak out. In my youth it was the Sex Pistols and the Clash - Holidays in the Sun, God Save the Queen, Know your Rights, White Riot. Check out the lyrics now and see how they resonate.

Anyway, my neighbour is the frontman Rock Star from the band I saw at Wembley stadium. He recently moved into what is obviously one of his many homes. He has quite clearly abandoned all he once sang about - maybe it's a lapse of reason, maybe not momentary, maybe the jabs have wiped that gene, who knows?

I first met him as he stepped out of his car, parked next to mine outside of his architectural spectacle. As a neighbour, the 'done thing' is to welcome him and introduce oneself with a handshake. 'Get away - Get away from me' he said, with fear in his eyes as if I were the next Mark Chapman approaching Lennon (how we need him around now). 'Six feet, six feet, Get Back!!' he cried. I had not given the 'safe distancing' bullshit a second thought, obviously not being a complier, it wasn't something I did, it was as irrational as getting jabbed with poison -who would do that? I guess there must have been a deep seated 'knowledge' that him, being a rock star, was also educated enough to know the stink of bullshit. But no, 'Safe distancing, Safe distancing' he barked.

Completely bamboozled, I scurried off muttering something about being a neighbour.

A week later, I was walking home, turned the corner to our lane and there was his big car, badly parked with one massive gull-wing door wide open. I had a little look in, as one does, and boy, does he like a mask!! There were packs and packs of them between front seats. At least he always has a fresh one, I thought, but he certainly was a big fan of re-breathing his CO_2. I thought he would pop out of his front door any minute so not wanting to be six, or any, feet near him, I carried on my way. 10 mins later, I emerged with my bin bags to see his door still wide open, like a massive black bird lopsided with injury. After disposing the bags in the big communal council bin, I thought I had best be that neighbour and remind him that his car door was wide open for all to see (and steal -those masks were pristine condition). So, ring the doorbell? yes, that's what one does. Worried, he now thinks I'm a stalker, I rang once and waited, no reply, after say 30 seconds, I rang again. 'What do you want?' his wife demanded. Err, I was thinking how to respond, 'What do you want?' she repeated. 'Your bloody car door is wide open', I said, like a teenager. 'It isn't', she said, 'It bloody well is', I said - I never use that word, usually just go straight to its big brother 'Fucking'. 'Have a look' I invited. Obviously, they could do so via one of the security cameras. 'Oh Gosh, sorry', she said, 'we're coming down, thanks.' Both appeared at the door with sheepish grins, 'I must have sat on the key fob', said the rock star.

I thought I should explain the manner in which I approached him on first meeting, 'Sorry, I just don't even think about this distancing stuff, it makes no sense'. The superstar frontman said, 'are you crazy, 150,000 people have died you know'. 'Well yeah, people die' I said, 'but no more burials and cremations than any other year, you don't really think they died of Covid do you?'. 'Of course, don't you watch the news? Don't you read the papers?? We're in the middle of a catastrophic pandemic'. 'So, where did the flu go this last year?' said I. 'Err, you are all mad around here', replied the man who taught me how to spot a fascist regime engaged in mass mind control before shutting his door, 'but thanks'.

Why don't rock bands do their job anymore? Well, it's no surprise when you look at Hollywood, Politicians, Media, Councillors and Educators - all heavily infiltrated and controlled to push their Marxist narrative, lies and propaganda. When the band that tells you, 'if you tolerate this, then your children will be next', denies entry to those who declined the death jab, you know something is very wrong.

I last spoke with my rock star neighbour when helping him discard his rubbish (no doubt 50% face nappies) into our big council bins. I offered the chance to continue our fascinating discussion, he said, 'Yes, maybe', with the look of someone thinking 'No, definitely not'.

Last I saw was that he reformed what was left of his supergroup, draping themselves in a massive blue and yellow flag singing some eastern European, some might say western Russian, folk song. A picture of four elderly gentlemen 'doing their charity bit for the BBC' at the local village hall.

Oh dear.

Substack 6

So, the aim of writing these episodes is that it will create a 'live feel' account of the 'end of times'. I know we are in a world war and for me and hundreds of thousands of others it has felt like it, day and night. No guns and bombs, not yet kinetic, but an information war involving two sides, good and evil. The Deep State (baddies) have infiltrated our societies over decades (in fact they are the Khazarians who have controlled us for centuries) to dilute our natural sense of danger, to divide, and then to conquer. They are doing a very good job, most people seem to be suffering a mix of Cognitive Dissonance and Stockholm Syndrome, dragging us all into the globalist's delightful Marxist offerings. However, I am also very aware of a good force that has infiltrated the other way using ancient Chinese military strategy, namely 'The art of war', penned by a chap named Sun Tzu. It's a complex but beautiful map of smoke and mirrors, appearing weak when strong and bad when good. It's the psyop division of the US military intelligence that has equally planned over decades, or more, a systematic destruction of the whole cabal, the swamp that will be drained. It involves the Ghost in the Machine - enjoy.

I have followed all of this very closely since watching Donald Trump getting attacked by endless assaults by the leftist woke brigade of liars and cheats, then to have a whole election blatantly stolen. I know that Q is a real US military psyop, a good psyop designed to confirm, retrospectively, that there is a plan in place to bring the cabal down, and to confirm each stage of the process. I also know that Devolution is in place. Once just a theory by Patel Patriot (John Herold), it is now very clear that Trump is still Commander in Chief of the military within a 'government in exile' following a declared foreign act of war. In-fact, two attacks from the CCP and others, a Bio-attack and a Cyber, election shifting, attack - including other domestic foes working for foreign powers- very clear acts of war.

The Patriots (the good guys) are so in control that they even made Biden unwittingly sign documents that kept the Executive Orders that created devolution in play - effectively signing his own death warrant.

So, it is now D-day +10, this is ten days since the Queen died. Tomorrow will be just about the only time that all of the deep state big wigs will be together under one roof. They can't excuse themselves and the event won't be cancelled. What an opportunity for something to happen. There have been many a time when I've been called a Qtard and a spreader of 'hopium' by other 'Truthers' (hate that term), and, yes, right now this evening of the 18th of Sept 2022, I am experiencing a little bit of hopium. Will they all get rounded up live on TV, like I hoped they would during Biden's illegitimate inauguration on Jan 20th, 2021? (didn't happen). Or will they all get letters falling out of their 'order of service' booklet telling them they are doomed imminently - as did happen at George Bush senior's funeral. I am sure something will happen, something. Everything is falling into place, The 'comm's' from the key Patriot players including Trump are ramping up to the storm. Of course, nothing actually happens as a prediction - if it did, it would be thwarted. That is not how it works, Q is the most amazing piece of work, on a par with the Bible or other religious blockbusters (rather it will be when viewed back in time, IMO). There comes a time when too many coincidences become impossible. It is utter genius.

I don't mind saying that as soon as I knew the Queen was ill and the family were travelling to her bedside, I became excited. Not because I am full of hate, but I knew from Q posts that the Queen needed to be removed before attacking the King - Check Mate. WWIII over! There have always been chess analogies and I have known the game was won some time ago, both sides were just playing out the remaining moves. I also knew that it was exactly 1776 (significant year of independence from the Crown - the head of the snake) days from the first Q post to the date of her death. There was also a post (3599) referring to harvest moon, which it was, six o'clock being dangerous, the 6 o'clock news broadcast the news of her death, there was a mention of the family being proud and Hunter becoming the hunted (MySonHunter, the film about Hunter Biden and 'the big guy', his Dad, being utterly corrupt paedophiles - as per the data on his laptop - released to the masses same day). That day, I was watching the clock and the news (on Telegram) wishing a 6 o'clock announcement. Tomorrow, the procession starts at 14:22 - why 2:22 pm? Why not 2:30? or 2:00 ??? it's not a bloody train. Also, King Charles (11:3 - count the alphabet), 11:3 being a major Q event mention, got all cross as his ceremonial pen leaked on him and another video showed further problems signing documents. Post 14:22 (time of procession) says 'Follow the Pen'. There are literally big 'match-ups' every week, and key comm's to confirm, the coincidences are too many.

This is how the mainstream media portray Q.

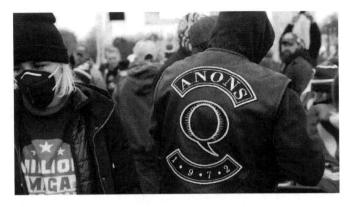

Anons, being some kind of Hell's Angel chapter. I'm so glad they don't understand it.

Anons merely work together to clarify messages from Q and decipher retrospectively - Q is a specialist US military intelligence group. Kash Patel, Devin Nunes and Dan Scavino Jr are very closely connected to Q. Donald Trump is the guy who acts as the bait - he is an absolute warrior.

Mainstream media always talks of Qanon (no such thing), which is a massive giveaway that they have no idea what it is or how it works - it's actually designed to stop the heavily armed Patriot civilians from rising up, creating the civil war that the deep state want. No wonder other 'Truthers' think of it as 'hopium'. They don't understand also, but they are focussed on other aspects of the resistance - we have all been working so hard for three years, losing friends and family, jobs, businesses, and masses amount of sleep!

I also know that October brings the storm to the deep state criminals and November, the mid-terms that will unanimously crush these evil liars and cheats - unless they nuke us first of course. October brings everything at once, Musk killing Twitter, exposing it as a manipulative brainwashing tool, SCOTUS returning to declare the 2020 elections illegal, Weiss killing the Bidens with Hunter's laptop evidence, Durham bringing down the FBI, Clintons and Obamas with the whole Russia, Russia, Russia treason and then the anti-globalist BRICS alliance outgrowing the Build Back Better's. Obviously, the baddies are going to throw everything at Trump now, they will try and indict him, they will try and cause a MAGA uprising, but it will be Antifa and BLM dressed as MAGA, as they did in the staged 'insurrection' on Jan 6th. They will create riots and then bring in the National Guard to try and close down the blue states to thwart the mid-terms. Good luck with that. Trouble is the 'normies' believe everything the MSM tell them, they have Trump Derangement Syndrome on top of their Cognitive Dissonance and their Stockholm Syndrome - their brains default to 'Orange Man Bad'.

So, tomorrow, I think I will watch and allow myself a hit of 'hopium' safe in the knowledge the storm is not quite due. Having said that, Trump is now playing WWG1WGA songs at his rallies with the distant but loud sound of increasing thunder and Putin just named his Falcon, Storm.

Pain.

Substack 7

I've not written anything here for around a year. I blame that on the beauty that is Twitter -or now 'X'.

X is a battleground, in fact THE battleground, it is where the good, the bad and the confused can debate, argue, insult and question. Until recently there never was such an open platform. The 'establishment' hate it. We know this now due to 'Twitter Files', the Post-Musk acquisition exposures of nefarious social media corruption - bots and algorithms hard wired into the Twitter platform (and all others) that created social engineering, 'The Thought Police', 'Nudge Units', 'Political Correctness', 'Virtue Signalling' and general Marxist 'Wokeness'.

Before this 'Digital Town Square' became available to all, we were unwittingly being silenced, quietly hidden, and pushed to the bottom of the chat lists if we spoke of narratives other than from the 'WEF Government's 'Ministries of Truth'. Society was being manipulated into a cycle of self-destruction, a whole set of 'isms created for new victims, hate was being created by messages of Anti-Hate, any attempt to swing even slightly back to a centre from an extreme left narrative would be swooped upon with cries of Far-Right Supremacists! Racists! Transphobic Nazis! and other over excited histrionics - more often than not, though, it was quietly hidden. It became clear via the 'Twitter Files' that the FBI and CIA, etc had been colluding with social media to ensure their 'social engineering' maintained support for the Cabal's nasty plans. Of course, the middle-class virtue signallers were never aware they were being so controlled - never aware they were just Turkeys voting for Christmas. The Commies always said they will conquer us without a bullet being fired.

Already I am noticing how many inverted commas are required when trying to sum up recent events, there is so much background and history to each element, it kinda proves the epic level of planning, time, detail and evil cunningness, this whole deep state operation required. Everything requires a deeper explanation - safe to say there will be a great encyclopaedia published after this period of hell with a handy index.

So, for the last year, since Elon walked into Twitter HQ carrying that sink (Let That Sink In - Q posts 621 & 4337, hmmmm?), I have been challenging the scientists, the politicians, the journalists and the doctors - and, well they don't like it up 'em do they?

Also, I have been compiling a Telegram channel designed to capture a chronological history of events from the perspective of 'we who are awake' or those actively working to counter official 'Government Science and Facts'. A selection of posts and memes. Hopefully, it will make an informative 'Killing Tyrants for Dummies' manual for future generations - should there be a remnant of Cabal beast left over for Agenda 83.

As I write, we have just witnessed an explosion of violence in Israel, and equally violent reprisals in Palestine - or so it seems. This initially looks like a false flag as there is no way Mossad or the IDF would not have known the attacks from Hamas were underway, or indeed being planned- their intelligence is known to be the best in the world. The attack happened on 7/10/23 and yet if we look almost exactly five years back, we see this:

Did they purposefully look the other way? Is this Israel's 9/11, are they going to use it as an excuse for an all-out attack on the likes of Iran? Is it a White Hat operation or set up by the Zionist Cabal? I have no idea right now but it certainly seems to be a second phase towards WW3, or the Big Scare Event (depending on which way you view things). In my opinion, if Taiwan is attacked by China soon, it will be the BSE, and Trump's allies are playing their roles perfectly.

Obviously, things are moving at such a pace, reading this back in even a few months may prove me to be tricked by a triple boomerang psyop!

So, what happened with my eternal mission to wake my brother up from his burning house? As previously written, a year and a half of sounding alarm bells, I got nothing but resistance, ridicule and argument from him - until 'Matt Le Tiss' popped up!

Suddenly he awoke with an apology - albeit two jabs late. Matt was famous and played football, so that obviously trumps a brothers' hard sourced evidence. All seemed well for a while, in fact celebrations were had. We, and my Son, were going to fight together from our WhatsApp trenches to beat the enemy - along with the legions of other digital warriors. We will share intel and science, identify targets, and hit them with truth bombs, I was so fired up.

That didn't happen though. Very quickly I realised it was only me mentioning 'The War', only me sending the latest intel, evidence of Vax Injury, Ukrainian Nazis, Biden's Crimes, Twitter Files etc. My brother started arguing back and my son completely ignored everything. I was being silenced by my own 'Brothers in Arms'.

This hurt. I was being gagged and I've never felt so much frustration, almost a betrayal. They just wanted to be 'Normies'. I was being sent pictures of happy families enjoying life while I was fighting to save our collective children's futures. At one point, to stir debate, I asked them this:

Which of the below do you guys expect our next generation to enjoy?

- To own a business
- To own a house
- To own land
- To own a car
- Rural / country life
- Travel / holidays
- Freedom to roam
- long life expectancy
- Farm crops / livestock
- Emigrate
- Have savings / accumulate wealth
- Have children
- Have grandchildren
- Access to fresh meat / veg / natural supplements
- Choice of medical treatment
- Good health
- Free speech
- Access factual education / information
- Freedom from conflict
- Ability to protect self & family
- To practice a religion
- Freedom for the pursuit of happiness
- To happily remain as the 'gender' they were born with

Maybe I was expecting too much, I mean they didn't sign up for adult education classes, but it seems like a good conversation opener. Anyhow, it was followed by the 'now boring' tumbleweed. Nothing. Just not going to engage.

I just couldn't bring myself to respond to their 'Normie' pics and comments, the big grins and the footy chat that came back after I shared something about Paedophilia, for example. They didn't see the juxtaposition. I needed to tell them that I was developing a big problem, that I was starting to feel some resentment to what was happening. It was making me ill. I couldn't stop trying to work out what to say, how to vent my boiling energy without permanently killing the relationships, especially with my son.

However, when I really analysed why they were keeping blinkers on, changing the subject, complaining of being too busy to read stuff, I knew it boiled down to them simply being Selfish and Cowardly. Not that they knew it, but ultimately, they were just hankering down, looking after their families, and not wanting to jeopardise their social and work relationships. Speaking out makes you lose friends and jobs. It does, it has happened to me and countless others - we are lucky because if you do it at Trump, Brand, Assange, Ballard and Tate level, you get a whole bunch of rape accusations and you will be found guilty by the fake news - front page for days.

I so wanted to tell them they were Selfish and Cowardly - in fact I did just that to my brother the other day but then went a step further.

Last week I stumbled across a link to a free site showing the film 'Sound of Freedom', I had not even gone that far with them, nowhere near the subject of child sex trafficking, but I sent it to them thinking it would be a good introduction and maybe even a new wake up call for the guys - after all it's about Children!! Naively, I imagined them sitting down to watch it with their wives and having one big OMG moment.

Instead, I had the mother of OMG moments! My brother responded with this, a hastily fumbled google search (I presume) led him to this from TIME magazine:

BY MEGAN MCCLUSKEYAUGUST 29, 2023 4:53 PM EDT

*Amid the hype over the cinematic double whammy of "Barbenheimer," another movie has crept up in the box office rankings this summer: **Sound of Freedom**.*

Directed and co-written by Alejandro Monteverde, Sound of Freedom is a low-budget action thriller about a U.S. federal agent who goes rogue on a mission to rescue children in Latin America from sex trafficking. Since its release on July 4, it's raked in over $180 million at the domestic box office, outperforming big-budget features like Mission: Impossible — Dead Reckoning Part One and Indiana Jones and the Dial of Destiny, and making it the highest-grossing indie film since 2019's Parasite.

*Billed as a story about the real-life Tim Ballard, a former special agent for the Department of Homeland Security and founder of the anti-trafficking group Operation Underground Railroad (O.U.R.), Sound of Freedom has become **mired in controversy over criticisms** that it features **misleading depictions** of child exploitation and **plays into right-wing conspiracy theories** associated with **the QAnon movement**. These associations have been perpetuated by both Ballard and his on-screen counterpart, Jim Caviezel, who has been a **prominent supporter of QAnon** for years.*

*The film's distributor, Angel Studios, has denied that Sound of Freedom is political or connected to **QAnon**. "Anybody who* watches this film knows that this film is not about conspiracy theories," Angel CEO Neal Harmon said in an interview. "It's not about politics."

While Sound of Freedom doesn't take a direct political stance or invoke **QAnon**, the fervent support for the film **from the right** has resulted it in being labelled "MAGA-friendly" and embraced by both mainstream conservatives and **far-right conspiracy theorists**. Former President **Donald Trump** recently hosted a screening of the film at his golf club in New Jersey, while Republican Senators Ted Cruz and Tim Scott have publicly praised it.

Much of the controversy surrounding Sound of Freedom stems from Caviezel and Ballard, who have openly supported **QAnon**.

Caviezel, best known for playing Jesus in Mel Gibson's The Passion of the Christ, has given speeches and interviews in which he promotes the **baseless conspiracy** theory that a **shadowy international cabal of top Democratic politicians and famous liberal elites are kidnapping children, forcing them into sex trafficking, and harvesting the chemical adrenochrome from their blood to consume as an elixir of youth.** The **conspiracy theory**, which has **anti-Semitic** roots, has been debunked numerous times by media outlets and scientific communities.

It is the most BS piece of propaganda I've read in a long while - I almost choked on it!

QANON, MAGA, Trump, Low Budget, Misleading Right-Wing Conspiracy Theories, Anti-Semitic - All highlighted in the first paragraph or two!

NB: all Cabal propaganda says QANON, whereas anyone who understands it knows there is no such thing, there is Q and there are Anons - anyone using the word QANON has absolutely no idea about it (odd because I spent the last 3 years sharing Q drops and their interpretations with my brother)

This unbelievable response from my brother was a seminal moment for me - I actually realised that he batted for the other team, and he always had. That explains three years of constant arguing and pushback. I thought he was just selfish and cowardly and had told him so but then I realised it was much more than that. He was completely stuck in his cycle of cognitive dissonance - 'The BBC are my friends', 'I trust my government', 'Orange Man Bad'… ….. etc, that he was always defending them. This means he is chained to a belief system and cannot escape it despite the truth slapping him the face with a wet fish. *(If I have used this phrase twice, sorry, I do like it)*

That now means I know I can't wake him up - it won't happen.

But this also means I am free from that overwhelming frustration, and I instantly feel lighter and healthier. In fact, after telling him he is batting for the wrong side, I also told him our battles are over - the three of us, no need for further discussion.

Let's get talking about football and music again - like the old days, it gives me some breathing space.

14. Part-time Punks

On the 1980 album Sandinista! by the British Punk band, The Clash, there was a track called 'Washington Bullets'. It was a politically charged song, as were a lot of theirs and several others of that time, but this seemed very well-educated and deep in detail. Most good Punk songs tended to be typically left leaning but honest. The lyrics took me to places my History teachers didn't, they sang about things like imperialist history, from the 1959 Cuban Revolution to the Nicaraguan Sandinistas of the 1980s, They mention the Bay of Pigs Invasion of 1961, the Dalai Lama, Salvador Allende and Víctor Jara, I knew the first but not the latter two, particularly folk musician, Jara's death at the hands of the Chilean military dictatorship in the actual stadium that now bears his name. It was mainly a criticism of the foreign policy of the United States but also references the treatment of pacifist Buddhist monks in the People's Republic of China during the Cultural Revolution and the Soviet Union's Invasion of Afghanistan.

I was sixteen when listening to this song, it was my first real introduction to historical events and issues around US foreign policy and Communism, it wasn't a punk song, more Calypso but it was a Punk band that also taught me that I went to school, where they 'teach you to be Thick'. Although I studied History, I knew nothing of any relevance, nothing that would help me in later life, and nothing that could help the society I was growing up in.

Joe Strummer, their frontman, also said: "I think people ought to know that we are ANTI-FASCIST, we're ANTI-VIOLENCE, we're ANTI-RACIST and we're PRO-CREATIVE. We're AGAINST IGNORANCE."

He had to say this because people were easily getting the wrong idea about their message, the exact opposite was creeping in – people are ignorant and easily led. This quote was very clear, well thought out, and it stuck with me despite the bullshit coming from the media and controlled Pop Culture.

Winding forward almost 40 years, I was invited to play with a Punk band, they needed a Drummer, and I was feeling the urge to get back behind a kit and to whack out my favourite three-chord wonders from the late Seventies. I met them in the Bass player's garage – we were a 'Garage Band' -perfect. A three-piece, the singer-guitarist looked the part – almost like he had typed in 'Full Punk Outfit' on his Amazon app.

We played several gigs, mainly in pubs, a few to shocked old ladies out for a quiet drink, and a few to large numbers of Punk fans – so mixed reactions. We also supported a couple of bands from the era, albeit only one grumpy original member who never developed a different income stream.

One gig was ridiculous, we had a different bass player who set the gig up. He was about 65 and looked like a surveyor. The 'crowd' wasn't - It was a table of his friends – all surveyors. No one else bar a couple of stray locals. We blasted out the set as best as we could, but it became painfully obvious the bass player knew the lines 30 years ago but had forgotten at least half. Bum note after bum note, it was awful, but Mr. Bass was rocking it, foot on his mates' table like a monitor, it was the four-stringed surveyor show – look at me, I use the word 'Fuck' at weekends. The singer, in his rent-a-punk outfit didn't seem to find anything wrong – I bloody did.

This was around Brexit time, I just couldn't stand watching the behaviour of the European MEP's and the shouty tearful, irrational, and over-emotional Labour opposition, both were trying all kinds of tactics to screw up, what I thought, the will of the people – albeit a small majority. Actually, I was originally anti-Brexit for two reasons; 1. I had only just returned from Portugal, where we lived happily for 15 years, 2. I thought it would be utter bloody chaos. However, intuitively I felt the behaviour and argument from the likes of Boris and Nigel were more 'honest' than their opposites. I have always said what I genuinely feel inside, not what people want to hear. I don't know why, because it can get me into trouble, but if you are true to yourself, you can sleep better at night – In my mind anyway.

I started to notice how the other band members were irrationally intolerant of people who didn't think like them, they thought what 'The Guardian' told them, I thought. They seemed to be very angry and hated anyone who didn't 'Think the Think'. I saw them look at each other and shake their heads in disapproval when I gave my opinion. I mean, am I allowed to have my own thoughts? We would bash out tunes enthusiastically to our audience barking at them as to how they should kick down authority, be true to themselves, go against the establishment, expose the liars, don't be fooled.

After one episode of mutual shaking heads in response to my misthinking during a practice session, I returned home to get a Facebook (yes, I was on that platform at the time – annoying people) message. 'Thanks for your time, we have found another Drummer' from the singer in the full punk outfit (Mohawk included with chin strap). Turns out he worked in a Bank by day.

I had been kicked out of the Punk band for being too, well, Punk.

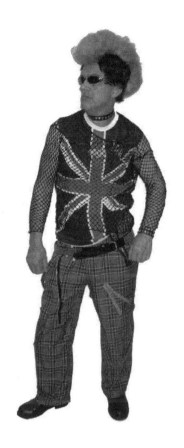

The bank clerk

15. No Debates Allowed

They ALWAYS resort to big shouty insults, rants without reply – my opinion is that they have no reply of any substance and that's why they won't debate, they can't debate because they have been programmed to react in only one way. Reactive stonewalling without anything originally proactive.

This is an example of the Semtex within the Brainwashed, minimal input, maximal output, this poor chap exploded into smithereens.

He was such a nice guy, often went to his house to watch our beloved Liverpool Football Club, we were part of a group with that in common. I have lost count of how many times we leaped into each other's arms, singing songs of pure red joy. The nights in the pub in collective nail-biting moments of despair, then elation. We loved each other, I know he thought my refusal to wear a mask in the pub was odd, considering I was the only one, and when forced to wear it while walking to the gents, I would simply hold it in my teeth, I noticed he didn't laugh like the others – nevertheless, we loved each other. We were Liverpool. He talked of being some kind of front-line hero, in the thick of it in some high drama emergency medical establishment, but I knew he was actually a care assistant at a local home for people with learning difficulties – difficult for him, yes but front-line superhero, I don't think. Anyway, everything was excused – we are Liverpool above all else - WWG1WGA (it's a Q thing – think the three musketeers).

Imagine how I almost inhaled my sausage when I saw this!!

Today

🔒 Messages and calls are end-to-end encrypted. No one outside of this chat, not even WhatsApp, can read or listen to them. Tap to learn more.

Am I reading it wrong or are you totally gone on the conspiracy shit? Hope I'm not right. Ed 20:33

I will happily debate this with you over a few hours ! As i said , if you guys don't want to hear my opinions then dont post stuff about US / UK politics or the virus because we probably won't agree . I totally agree that we should stick to footy topics in the group. 20:49

No debate as we have nothing in common.

I've been working non stop since

No debate as we have nothing in common.

I've been working non stop since March with friends who are on their fucking knees. That's my reference point.

You've been busy felling sorry for your fucking self with too much time on your hands masterbating to David Icke podcasts!

Go fuck your self

Ps- you really don't understand what Liverpool really is. Was it the colour of the jersey!!!!!!! 20:58

nice and rather presumptuous

21:01

You've been busy felling sorry for your fucking self with too much time on your hands masterbating to David Icke podcasts!

Go fuck your self

Ps- you really don't understand what Liverpool really is. Was it the colour of the jersey!!!!!!!

20:58

nice 👍 and rather presumptuous

21:01

You were your selfishness on your sleeve. Let's see if you call the nhs if you or yours are in trouble. No assumptions- only you will be placed to answer that.

21:06

enough said mate - still far too presumptuous to warrant a reply

21:08

He's utterly beside himself with rage, can't spell with anger, vitriol coming out of his ears. I laughed so loud. Apparently, I didn't know what Liverpool really was! What IS Liverpool, I mused. What really IS it?

I thought I would share with the group. 'Hey, guys, does anyone know what Liverpool is?', I just don't really understand apparently'. They just thought I wanted a deep philosophical debate, didn't get any takers, a few emoji's but my NHS superhero must have seen it. He must have seethed. I hope so anyway.

I thought it a very nice offer to debate something important – surely there are two sides to every story? - but they just can't seem to do it, can they?

They won't do it on Twitter (X), just a barrage of abuse and insults. These people have been bred, or certainly socially engineered.

Now for The School Dad's. A 'boy band' of about 18 wet beardy, top-knot haired, woke as hell, bit dull, 'my Toby this and my Jacob that', brigade. I knew a couple before the staged COVID nonsense, one I liked, he was a bit shy but harmless and reminded me of my old and best friend Matt whom I went to Israel with, who sadly died a few years ago.

They had 'drinks night' every other Tuesday, allowing a good thirteen days to recover. Obviously not much else happened for them, so they were always super excited, laughing too enthusiastically and always happy to jump right into reminding us all of the latest cause we all needed to be aware of.

I went to one, just before they collectively felt it was all too irresponsible to meet in the light of government advice – pre-mandates, and they all seemed so amazed that I played in a Punk band at night while in the medical profession by day. 'Amazing' they kept saying, Amazing. I was invited into their WhatsApp group 'Man Drinks - Pub' – must have taken some thought. I also thought the word 'Man' was a bit debatable - call me old-fashioned.

Several months later after weeks of unbearable drop-off mornings and pick-up evenings outside the school gates, me being the only unmasked, getting hard stares from people I used to converse with, and me giving hard stares back, this happened! AMAZING!!!

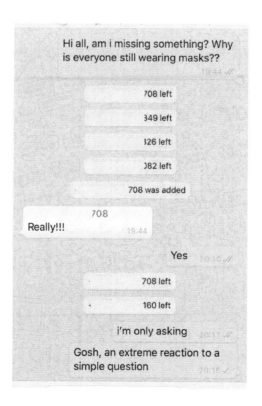

It takes a while for it to sink in.

One nicely asked, innocent question and BANG, BANG, BANG, BANG, BANG, BANG – a mass evacuation, instant bailout. What really makes me laugh is the first to jump, quietly creeps a toe back in to ask "Really!!!" – was it a question? I'm not sure now, no question marks but exclamation marks (like a proper English middle-class lady from the fifties reacting to perceived rudeness) – I just love how he waited for my "yes" answer, reaffirming my original question, before instantly jumping out again.

Like the 'slightly more' brave puppy in a litter, 'OK, boys cover me I'm going in – oh shit, no, sorry, I mean no harm'.

Then another jumps – while I'm not looking. I felt invincible, like King Dong, what power!!

They really, really don't want a debate.

16. It wasn't me, it was my Strawman, your honour

Finding out about how we have been stripped of our sovereignty with the cunningness of Maritime Law was a new depth of discovery for me. How we have all been tricked into surrendering our inalienable rights, or believing we don't have them, for us to have little knowledge of the Magna Carta and the Bill of Rights, is the biggest of all crimes against humanity. To replace common law, the law of the land with one of the waters, is to trick us all into signing away our rights. We are conned, on a daily basis, into signing away our rights. Words with double meanings, the capitalisation of your name to denote a corporation that someone else can own – your Strawman. Common law is very much worth studying, it is complex but a real jaw-dropper when you understand it, a bit like when it clicks how the Private Western Banks operate their Fiat system, the illusion of 'money'.

That was a very basic summary and here is my experience of it.

We received our 'summons' from the council, obviously not the court itself. I say obviously because we were primed. We knew that if the council decided to push you to their limit, to pay supposedly outstanding taxes, they would send you a 'summons'. It would indicate the letter came from the court as a real summons should, but the letter has no seal nor official signature from the clerk of the court, in fact, it would be signed from the council. We knew it was a scam in advance.

We, my wife and I, arrived at the court on the day of the

'hearing' to find ourselves herded into a wing along with maybe 100 other council tax 'defendants'. Coincidently, they want you to believe, all 100 or so all had the same hearing date, all of us were going to appear on the same day. Individual court hearings in one day for 100 defendants? Either it was a massive court with many courtrooms, or each of us would get five minutes and it would last nine hours non-stop. We knew, however, that the council had actually hired a large area within the court building because they wanted to scare you into making a deal 'to prevent the imminent court action'.

We took our ticket number and sat with the hundreds of poor souls who were clearly struggling with the hell that is modern life. Most were good, honest people simply drowning under the taxes dumped on them – or their strawman.

We watched them being led into cubicles by council workers, trained to smile as they rob you. We heard them very kindly offering a way out of the punishments hiding around the corner. Jail, Bankruptcy? It certainly wasn't going to be nice. So, we heard people saying a lot of 'pleases and thank-you's' as they were signing up to unaffordable payment plans, before they made an exit in haste, closely avoiding the guillotine.

We approached one of the head council officers and said we were summonsed to appear in court so that's what we wanted to do. 'I beg your pardon' she said 'No, you don't want to do that, let's see how we can prevent that. 'Er, no, we have been asked to appear before the magistrates, so that's what we must do, it says so here on their 'summons', we said. We were passed up to a more senior chap, one without a friendly first name badge. The council tried several times to persuade us that we could come to an arrangement with them to avoid facing the magistrates.

We said there is no arrangement to be had as we do not owe anything so we will wait to be seen by the magistrates. We were eventually led to a waiting area. One other person was there, a Polish lady, who didn't understand what was going on. The other 98 were all exiting with new debt, they just signed up for.

After a couple of hours, the court usher invited us into the court. Exciting and slightly terrifying. We talked over what we were advised to do, no not make joinder, do not agree to anything. We have the power and are in control. We had prepared ourselves to not sit or stand as asked when the magistrates enter, so if we are led in and asked to sit, we won't then stand when asked to when the magistrates walk in, or if we are standing and the magistrates say, 'please be seated', we will remain standing. Then we would assertively ask the magistrates if they were acting under their oath of office today.

Our expectations from the course we attended were that as soon as the magistrates heard those dreaded words, they would about turn, leave the courtroom and we would then declare the court adjourned. Simple.

When we entered, we were informed that the magistrates were busy behind the court in a meeting and the court clerk addressed us asking if we were there to A. contest the amount or B. discuss a payment arrangement. Obviously, we said neither and that we wanted to see the magistrates as we were summonsed.

We were given the sternest of stern looks and told they were busy, 'not possible right now', and led back outside to wait, before doing so we declared that we needed to be seen and heard before 2 pm as we had childcare issues. Our court time in the letter was set for 10 am sharp. We sat and waited for another couple of hours. Just after 1 pm we were informed by the usher that the magistrates had adjourned for lunch and would not be back until well after 2 pm!! Wow, they're scared of us, they've run off! We laughed.

We were then approached by the council chap without the name tag who told us they will reschedule for us in a couple of months and then suddenly, and surprisingly went into a monologue about him being 'under oath whist on the court premises'. This was unprompted, although it came after we asked for his name and job position. We left shaking our heads feeling very empowered.

The next day we received emails from him saying how nice it was to meet us and that they would get back to us about rescheduling.

We waited a good few months expecting to get called again. This time we didn't receive a summons but an email confirming the new court date. Lots of people offered their advice during this time, one suggested a 'cease and desist' letter, we had considered that but chose a 'subject access request' to confirm records the court held on us. We were in a combative mood. Probably unwisely. The reply was disappointing, something about it being the wrong department, so maybe our fault there – not researching the right recipient.

Anyway, we turned up at the court, expecting the same situation where the council staff would try and get us to agree on a deal. We had sought further advice and hatched a plan that would incriminate all involved with this next process.

We were pre-prepared with home-printed formal notices, complex legal history, and areas for all council staff to be named, and for them to sign, acknowledging their participation. They won't want to go there. They did.

The letters:

'On 21 July 1993, the then Speaker of The House of Commons, Betty Boothroyd, issued a reminder to the courts. She said: "There has of course been no amendment to The Bill of Rights... the House is entitled to expect that The Bill of Rights will be fully respected by all those appearing before the courts." There is a provision in the Bill of Rights Act 1688/9 which states: 'That all grants and promises of fines and forfeitures of a particular person before conviction are illegal and void.' This states that a conviction is necessary before a fine or forfeit can be imposed.

As you will be aware, the Bill of Rights is a "constitutional statute" and may not be repealed impliedly. This was stated in the case Thoburn v City of Sunderland, the decision commonly referred to as the 'Metric Martyrs' Judgement. This was handed down in the Divisional Court (18 February 2002) by Lord Justice Laws and Mr Justice Crane. Copy if the Judgement can be provided, however, to paraphrase the judgment's relevant sections 62 and 63. 62. 'We should recognise a hierarchy of Acts of Parliament: as it were "ordinary" statutes and "constitutional statutes." The special status of constitutional statutes follows the special status of constitutional rights. Examples are the... Bill of Rights 1688/9...' 63. 'Ordinary statutes may be impliedly repealed. Constitutional statutes may not...' This was upheld by Lords Bingham, Scott, and Steyn in an appeal that went to the House of Lords on Monday 15

July 2002. It is therefore settled in law that without a conviction in a properly convened court, any fine or forfeiture issued prior to conviction is <u>illegal and void</u>. What that means is there can be no fine or forfeiture without conviction before a jury of one's peers. This is a <u>fact in law and irrefutable</u>.

Further, it is our understanding that The Local Government Finance Act 1992 and its accompanying Regulations, enable the Council to use a Magistrates Court, which is an Administrative Court (Private bar Guild Tribunal, NOT a public court of record), to obtain a Liability Order against any 'person' the council believes to be in breach of the LGFA 1992. An act that solely derives limited delegated authority to the VOA and local authorities (councils) on the basis of 'prescribed'. Your legal team should understand the concept of 'prescribed' and the liability that therefore places on the individuals (You Mr/Mrs) at the council trying to enforce the LGFA 1988, 1992. Halesbury's laws of parliament, states, no administrative court can be legitimised because of the constraints on the Monarch's oath - Coronation Oath Act 1688, being Constitutional Law.

Given the facts expressed above please answer the following:

1) Does the Local Government Finance Act 1992 and its accompanying regulations Supersede Constitutional Statutes?

2) By ignoring this notice and allowing any form of enforcement of the Local Government Finance Act 1992, would you, in your personal capacity, be guilty of the offences listed in Archbold (Criminal Pleading Evidence & Practice) section 1 - 6, Disobedience to Statutes?

3) Can the named individual(s) at the Council please provide me

with the necessary information regarding their public, professional indemnity insurances should I need to take civil and criminal action against them.

4) Are the named individual(s) aware that their pursued authority is derived unequivocally on the basis of 'prescribed' and what that therefore means in terms of liability?

We were left until the last case for the morning, we were in the same waiting room as the Council staff, sat at opposite ends, they had their papers with them, our papers that they appear to have signed- worryingly.

They were led into the court and stayed there a good 30 minutes before we joined them.

We were then asked to go into the courtroom and were led to some pews behind the council officers. As primed, we were expecting magistrates to walk in, then we would do the opposite to their sit/stand request, and ask to see their oaths etc, then they walk out, and we leave. We had gone through this several times at home and practiced in the car on the way.

But no! When we entered there was a Judge sat there! A Judge? He introduced himself, seemed like a nice chap, quite friendly, please take a seat, he said. 'No, we're ok thanks, I said, with wobbly confidence. I pounced and interrupted whatever he was about to say, there were around 30 people in the room, I had no idea of their roles. "Are you acting under your oath of office"? He confidently said 'yes', he was. He then said, "I could go and get it and show you if you like," I declined, my wheels were falling off. Hold on, none of this was supposed to happen, 'where are the fucking magistrates, why didn't they show up, with their bogus authority?' I thought.

Then he said our letters were very good and true in many places but ultimately didn't prevent the council from charging us council tax to pay for local services. At this point, we were stumped. Nothing was going to script. I felt like a smart arse at school being shamed for being a twat. Everyone in the classroom thought I was a twat. I thought I was a twat.

Maybe I would just slip back into mindless compliance to work, without complaint and pay my never-ending taxes, become beholden to my Tax Identification Number, (TIN), be that Tin Man – 'if I only had a heart' – but I do, somewhere.

So, being completely disarmed and my pants pulled down, I offered mitigating circumstances as to why we couldn't afford it, redundancy due to lockdowns, my daughter's expensive mental health treatment, my mental health, the cat's anxiety issues – anything and everything. He was sympathetic, genuinely, and he told the council officers to stand before him, they did.

Yes, we have to pay, but only in affordable instalments, even if it takes years, he told them. So almost certainly we have now made contract with them and agree to the monies 'owed' but will push it down to as little over £0 per month as possible, quoting what the judge ordered.

Not wanting to tempt fate, but we always seem to slip to the bottom of their priority list as we are still awaiting our deal over a year later.

Maybe we did rattle things.

Next up – This is the bit that will either age very well, or embarrassingly bad.

Nevertheless, this is where I hang my hat - with confidence.

The next three chapters are my summaries of a very complex counter offensive.

17. Orange Man Bad

"Today's ceremony, [however], has very special meaning because, today, we are not merely transferring power from one administration to another or from one party to another, but we are transferring power from Washington, D.C., and giving it back to you, the people."

January 2017 President Donald Trump's Inauguration Speech

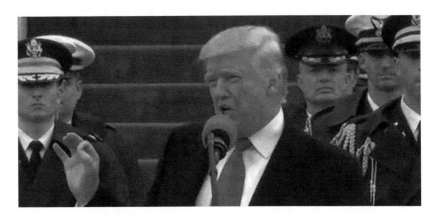

Who actually paid attention to what was said? Listening to the whole speech now sends shivers down my spine – clearly, and for the first time since JFK, a man was bravely taking down the whole Deep State – the worldwide enemy of the people. Very few people realise this.

In the next few chapters I will reveal just how significant the military men flanking him are – here's a clue, 'Hats'. You really think he could, or would want to, do all of this alone?

The 45th and last President of the United States, I heard this said back in 2016. I really thought it was prophetic, The Last! I listened to those saying he will cause WWIII, collapse the economy and, by the way, he is a racist misogynist. I listened and was horrified when he won. I just thought he would be worse than all that had come before, all the warmongers, the liars, the Blairs and Bushes and Clintons. I was always aware of how they all ended up doing bad things. I was always aware there was a Uni-party - Labour / Conservative, or Democrat / Republican – always sounding so fresh and promising but all ending up doing exactly the same, the cost of living goes up, wars are created, homelessness grows, as does crime – the people always suffered. The rich got richer.

I knew deep down we were lied to regarding 9/11, I knew instinctively building 7 was demolished and a plane didn't hit the Pentagon, I knew they made up the Weapons of Mass Destruction, I knew Dr Kelly didn't kill himself. I knew there was a Military Industrial Complex before I heard the term. I knew they were at pains to paint Russia as some persistent evil threat, I started to listen to some of the things Putin was telling us (The people of the West) and they just seemed more believable than Blair, Bush, Obama, or the BBC. Russia was due to stage the world cup in 2018 and the reports were, 'do not go, you will be killed, The Russians are Nazi thugs – it's in their nature, hard-wired'. This just seemed so desperately reported, I never really studied history, but I was sure Russia was our ally against Hitler in the last war.

Without joining any dots and without any deep diving, I had a suspicion of an 'Axis of Evil', running right through Washington, I knew the CIA created colour revolutions in other countries, also as a teenager, I had a very strong fear of Catholicism, all religion in fact, but the Catholic Church scared the crap out of me, The

Pope just seemed wrong – the song by The Damned, Anti-Pope, resonated with me so much in the late 1970's – check it out man! The Vatican seemed to ooze very bad 'vibes', sinister, and then The City of London, the financial capital of the world, seemed closed, cold, and self-serving. I never joined the dots but there must have been some little voice in me suggesting I should – that came years later.

For a few weeks, I thought Donald J Trump was a racist liar, an evil crook. I was supposed to think like this, of course. I thought he was part of the upper tiers of that triangle, the one with the eye at the top, didn't really understand the components of the Triangle but that eye looked scary, Trump was scary.

Then he said he wanted to sit with Putin and share a burger, he would also go and have a chat with Kim Jong-un. OK, that's different, I thought, not the usual combative threats to Russia, Iran, North Korea, and the other evil baddies with nukes. No, he wanted to sit and have a chat. Just talk things through.

'Art of the Deal', the name of his bestseller book, I had not read it but understood it offers great insight. He was the best at bringing together two parties with their own vested interests, often miles apart initially, then coming together with both feeling they have achieved their key aims. Maybe both thinking they were the winners. 'Isn't that exactly what the world needs right now?', I thought back then (and almost eight years on the same thought prevails!) Also, here was a man who was already a multi-millionaire, unlike the career politicians, he was different – a businessman. Take a look at those on Capitol Hill, or Westminster, they have £100k salaries or so, very modest compared to high-level businessmen, probably not even enough to maintain a whole family, but enough to allow those who wish to serve their country and their fellow countryfolk. Serve with honesty and represent your constituents, do it for a few years, then get back into work, or live off it from then on, write a book, give after-dinner speeches, serve on company boards honourably. But no, they are all multimillionaires, how? How do they enter politics with a net worth of a few hundred thousand bucks and within a few years a zero or two is added, how does that happen? Corruption, backhanders, money for lobbying, votes, and policies, that's how. They become sick with greed and power, they become beholden to corporations, foreign regimes, or billionaire psychopaths, they get caught up in evil, get up to no good, and then live under the constant threat of 'Kompromat', they become puppets. They become owned.

Clearly, this was a guy who didn't need to be bought.

This was the man who would cause WWIII and collapse the economy – or so Democrats and Media told us. In fact, he was the only President not to start a war for far longer than I could remember, and the economy rocked. Near the end of his first term (yes, there are more), he had brought peace to the Middle East and pretty much stopped millions of illegal immigrants from 'invading' the country unchecked.

So, what happened, and why does everyone hate him? In the UK, my little survey to 'litmus test' the levels of Awake, revealed a 95% strong dislike of Donald Trump, regardless of their Awake / Asleep status. Even when I showed the picture of Biden, people said, 'ooh not sure, but better than that idiot before him'. They really do not like him, how could they with images of the Trump

Barrage Balloon in nappies flown in London by radical Mayor Khan? They remember him holding Teresa May's hand while descending a slope, they remember him advising us to drink bleach for Covid, they remember him talking of grabbing pussies, and they assume he is a racist and are currently watching him jumping from court to court defending any kind of 'crime' the corrupt and radical left in the US can 'Trump Up'.

A constant wave of attacks from all sides from day one, riots, accusations, Impeachments and then Covid – he had so much to deal with that nobody saw who he really was, and what he was prevented from doing. Clearly, his presidency was constantly being sabotaged by dark forces.

The more they attacked him, the more I liked him. I started to tell people but couldn't find anyone agreeing with me, My Mother announced, on behalf of both parents, "We don't like Trump," as if it were some kind of a well-thought-out final assessment after a thorough examination of his administration's actual policies. As if they were any different from everyone in their neck of the woods. "Congratulations Mum, you're supposed to not like him," I said, knowing full well it was a clear case of 'Trump Derangement Syndrome'.

Everyone I knew had it, (TDS), they didn't like him at all but could never really articulate why. They had been so indoctrinated into hating him and so manipulated by the drip feed media that their brains just go 'ORANGE MAN - BAD', on sight. If they were Cats, they would be on all fours in an inverted 'U' with fully erect back hair and a massive bush tail, immediately. 'Orange Man Bad', like a reflex, doesn't even enter the brain, a single synapse from sensory to motor – they have no choice or control – it just happens.

My interracial marriage and mixed-race kids give me a pass. I am allowed, to a certain extent, to have some wider opinions and insight. My wife was always one step ahead of me regarding being awake to the nefarious elite, I remember a few years back, her asking me, "so, what do you think about Bill Gates?" I said, naively, "I guess he is just a philanthropist, wanting to help us all, leave his mark as a good man before departing" – she just laughed in a very patronising way, and of course she had every right to. But she didn't like Trump and was a tad pissed off with me saying I did, she even had suspicions of a deep-seated and previously hidden racism within me.

I started to openly support him on Facebook (before I closed my account) and, 'Man did I get a torrent', most people thought I was joking but a very old friend decided I needed a lecture. He lived in the US, so obviously thought that meant he knew more. He literally told me Trump was coming after my wife and kids, he was so racist, he wanted them eradicated and my supporting him would only hasten that fate.

Immediately after my wife watched the Q-based movie, Plan to Save the World (more on this later), she became a very strong Trump supporter. It was her 'AHA Experience' on this side of things.

Moving towards the end of 2020, I was telling everyone, Trump HAS to win this election, or we will get TYRANNY – to what degree, I didn't know exactly, but I knew it would be bad, very bad.

We knew the media were falsely claiming Joe Biden was ahead in the polls running up to the 2020 election, it was obvious, twenty people attended his rallies - when he did them - all 20 stood in their allotted Covid circles and occasionally clapped – if they could understand when they should. Twenty Thousand attended Trump's. Or more. Clearly, he was by far the most popular candidate. Biden was a mumbling geriatric and his son's laptop revealed a lot of bad, incriminating stuff – they were saying it was a Russian Setup – but we knew different, even in the UK. My wife and I placed a bet on a Trump victory, 30/1, £100 each, we were already planning our £6K shopping spree.

The night of November 3rd going into the early hours of the 4th was a total shocker. All was going well for the world and humanity, Trump was leading consistently, and then we saw it – FLIP! A few thousand votes jumped from Trump to Biden, exactly the same volume, live on one of the US TV channels, then they stopped counting, or they closed voting centres due to 'burst pipes'- anything. We later saw hundreds of people filing into to other voting centres laden with heavy bags, shopping bags, leather holdalls, suitcases at 3.30 AM, then we saw clear vertical jumps in the blue line – impossible, live votes worming along somewhere between a horizontal 'time' axis and a vertical 'number' axis, impossible. It was impossible for a sheer vertical line without it being a massive dump. Then FOX called it, Biden had bloody won. Fuck.

It was a fix, we were instantly concerned about the future of the world, and our £6K.

Knowing you have just watched a banana republic style election fix in the USA was more troubling than I can explain. Probably the same as your football team getting cheated out of a victory, finding out your wife is sleeping with your best mate, and being told you have cancer – in one five-minute blast.

The insurrection occurred on November 3rd, 2020, not January 6th, 2021.

I could write so much about his first term but really need to focus on why I say 'first'.

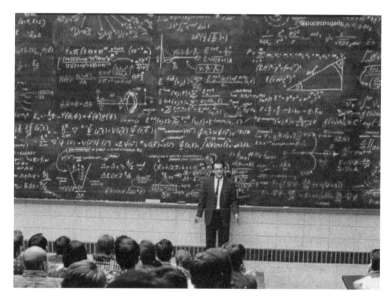

Me trying to explain the next two chapters – wish me luck.

18. Q

I remember seeing a grainy video of Jerome Corsi speaking about Trump. He looked like a bullfrog in a suit, but somehow trustworthy. This would have been before he got caught up in the 'Russia, Russia, Russia' collusion witch hunt by special counsel, Robert Mueller – now completely proven as largely concocted and 'made up' by the people around Hillary Clinton, involving the infamous (Christopher) 'Steele dossier'. They do that though, don't they, anyone revealing anything they don't want revealing gets hauled into some dodgy 'scandal'.

Corsi spoke of being informed by some top military generals that they were planning a military coup d'état, to remove the Obama administration by force. For some reason he was subsequently informed that they had changed their plans and had persuaded Donald Trump to stand for President, and for him to work with them and their special intelligence operators in a coordinated plan to bring down the entire Deep State, once and for all. A Military Coup was very risky and would not be tolerated by the world's media and foreign governments, a lot of whom were controlled by the 'enemy'. The Generals would help ensure he is elected – they knew even then that the elections would be tampered with - and Military Intelligence would set up a cyphered system to communicate the existence of their 'White Hat' plan while it was being carried out – they knew it was a long-haul plan with risks. They had just one opportunity to get it right and they needed to avoid a civil war - that would be the biggest risk.

Corsi, you will read on Google, was a known 'conspiracy theorist' and involved with Info-Wars and the likes of Alex Jones – who was recently fined over $900 Million for questioning aspects of a mass shooting. 'QAnon', as it was called by the media, was a 'cult', or so I thought. It had the chap in the Guy Fawkes Mask, appearing in grainy videos like he was interrupting mainstream TV. Otherwise known as 'V', for Operation Vendetta, and the Million Mask March in 2015 with the 'hacktivist' group called 'Anonymous' – a growing resistance, against the establishment, movement - all very thought-provoking, while the stuff of comic books. Hero/Anti-hero? Interesting.

For some reason, I thought it was fascinating, and I hate science fiction. I decided to investigate.

Key moments for me were when Trump was surrounded by all the top US military generals, the real ones we didn't see on TV, and their wives, roughly 30 of them, aligned for the cameras. He said to the press, quietly "What you are witnessing is the calm before the storm." "What storm Mr President?" asked an intrigued female reporter. "You'll find out," came the confident response and a lot of knowing smiles from the assembled group.

I managed to access the channels used by 'Q', set up by Ron Watkins, called 8kun, or copies of such made available to people like me scrabbling around the internet in the UK, and tried to make sense of the messages and questions posed by the 'Anons', nothing really did. But it seemed BIG and way too complex for any hoax.

I watched the film 'Plan to Save the World' by Joe M – it's currently on Rumble and I would recommend it to anyone who isn't aware of this side of 'awakeness'. It made me very confident there are some good people who have come together, with clout, to take control of the world and free the people from the evil elite. This went back a long way in planning, some point at evidence of it even while JFK was still alive.

It made total sense. I was led to further information, describing how Trump built up what is called a 'White Hat' alliance of world leaders during his world 'Capitulation Tour', pretty much immediately after taking office. He was supported by a military plan, and decades in its planning, he was armed with incredibly incriminating evidence, horrible stuff I won't go into – DECLASS, this was declassified military intelligence information, millions of gigabytes of evidence taken from phones, computers, and servers, digitally, by cutting edge surveillance methods, they only had one slim opportunity to get all this, and it was enough to bring all corrupt leaders and Deep-State players down - unless they cooperated.

First, he went to Saudi Arabia, where he was given the 'ceremony of the sword', only ever afforded to the highest king of the kingdom – all Muslim leaders were in attendance, and they all agreed on a complete peace plan to eradicate extremist ideology after listening, like naughty school children, to their new headmaster, who simply won't tolerate their crap. He then visited Israel, The Palestinian National Authority in Bethlehem, The Vatican City, Brussels (Belgium), Italy, Poland, Germany, France, Japan, South Korea, China, Vietnam, The Philippines, Canada, Singapore, Guam, and ending up in the UK where the Queen famously stopped to let him walk ahead of her - in an apparent act of submission.

The plan was – and remains – to take down the cabal, it is a plan to replace the evil with the good. It involves the biggest sting operation imaginable. The Deep State players were drawn into an information war, that they will lose. It is a battle, so meticulously planned that it is already won, but both sides will play out the final chess moves. It will get increasingly nasty as the end gets nearer for the Cabal, the Mafia, and their minions.

Trump and the Generals interrupted a sixteen-year plan, 2 x Obama followed by 2 x H. Clinton terms, they were going to bring in the WEF's Agenda 30 with stealth, long drawn-out pandemics, and collapsing economies, starvation, and war, before finally offering a (deadly) vaccine that all would welcome. Sounds a bit far-fetched to some, but evidence of this is wide-ranging, the cabal and satanic 'evildoers' (Bush-Speak) have not exactly hidden their plans. Signalling and symbolism seem to be their modus operandi. 'Operation Warp Speed' was designed to compress this, eliminating the stealth. With this interruption and the clear threat of a second term in 2024, the deep state had 4 years to accelerate everything – this is where they would be exposed, they would be out of the shadows, the people will see clearly what their agenda is and 'rise up'. The alliance and the other good guy players, such as those BRICS nations (note the R and the C) will play their part in the fall of the cabal. A gold-backed currency to kill the (petro) dollar. Follow the yellow brick road.

Meanwhile, they will throw everything at the Patriots and the MAGA movement, and they will try to create a civil war to disrupt the plan. They will fill countries with illegal immigrants, unchecked - a good time to be reminded of Trump's 2022 speech where he recited 'The Snake' poem. They will trigger a vision of Hell. 80+ million Patriots, heavily armed, will naturally want to fight back, you have to keep them 'at-ease', 'hold the forking line', 'Trust - The - Plan'.

My wife and I used to laugh at old Charlton Heston, bless him, telling the NRA conference how they would need to 'prise his gun from his cold dead hands', hilarious! Chaz, mate, you're not in a movie now, calm down – I mean as if your government would ever become tyrannical! Eeek!

I won't go into any detail about any of the 'mass shooting' events in the US over the last decade or so, but I will say that I believe a portion of them are False Flag events – not to say they didn't happen, but I do believe they were 'facilitated'. They want to disarm the people. The 2nd amendment is the main obstacle preventing tyranny from just 'steam-rollering' in. Look at the Police in Australia, or the UK, where governments took away the people's right to bear arms, look at how they very quickly acted for the tyrants – the Flying Monkeys.

There will be multiple False Flag events, a tried and tested communist tactic - and they will do everything in their power to bring down Trump – including imprisoning him, or worse.

However, think this; – The Presidents Precedents. Everything they are trying to do to him, an 'ex' President, opens the door for the same thing back against all deep state players – including former Presidents – Bush, Clinton, Obama, Biden. This, so far, includes looking at all bank accounts of not only the President but their families and any businesses they are associated with. It includes official documents they hold; it means the FBI can carry out dawn raids, they can arrest and take mug shots, they can dig up any 'sexual crimes' from the past, I could go on.

The facts are, the corrupt radical left justice system, which took years to infiltrate, will always struggle to find real dirt, real evidence. The latest involves Trump over-valuing property to get a loan from a bank, the loan was fully repaid, with interest, on time, and the bank has no issues (banks do their own due diligence with loans, it's up to them to evaluate the customer's ability to pay back). It's a pathetic attempt to lock him up. They all are because he is clean. Does anyone think the White Hats would spend 60 years planning the biggest mafia takedown in history by allowing their key player to be compromised? No, they wouldn't. They would have had that more than covered.

> **"In reality, they're not after me, they are after you,**
> **I am just in their way."**
> **"I gladly take all the slings and all the**
> **arrows for you, the people"**
> **DJT**

The Plan, Trust the Plan.

This is the whole point of Q. The plan will take a long time and be very difficult, there will be moves and counter moves, smoke and mirrors, people will likely take matters into their own hands and rise up against the Biden regime, there is a danger of a civil war and that would kill the plan. It would mean going back to the military coup.

They eventually decided to let Biden steal the election of 2020. While they stole it, all incriminating data was collated. They 'caught them all' as Trump declared, and Space Force has the evidence.

The United States Space Force - sounds like Star Trek fiction, but very real, a branch of Military Intelligence set up by Trump – A lone military force that can bypass the normal judicial system and provide evidence against civilians, avoiding the 'Posse Comitatus Act' that otherwise prevents this. Every single Digital 'Bit' of evidence, they were ready and waiting, and they intercepted it all, even the Direct Messages within Twitter, where they thought they had their safe house, or sharing a Gmail account and communicating in 'Drafts'. Epstein also had them all, compromised, in his little black book, secretly filmed even, the globalists controlled their players with the threat of exposure, but they were all in the club – just couldn't help themselves – addicted to something demonic, I care not to go into.

This is the biggest sting operation ever, working its way to the inevitable end.

Nothing Can Stop What Is Coming. The Storm. Pain.

In my opinion, Q is the most exquisitely executed military intelligence operation in history. It obviously involved decades of planning and the most elaborate algorithms, generated by the most powerful Quantum computers designed by the most brilliant minds. Bletchley Parks' big brother.

'So, how does Q work, is it 'some kind of Nostradamus'? Most people ask.

Actually, it is used retrospectively to provide evidence that the plan is on track and unfurling as expected. Trust the Plan. No, don't just sit back and wait to be saved – you have work to do!

Q posted 4966 messages from Oct 28th, 2017, ending on Nov 27th, 2022, with a massive gap from Dec 2020 to June 24th, 2022, with only 13 posts following. No more are necessary, everything is covered. Everything is and has been rolling out to plan – massive events, almost daily, and all since 'Biden' 'took office' (consecutive inverted commas for a reason, both are more than debatable). All events feature in the Q posts.

I will only go so far as to say, that there are known people who create 'comms', these are hidden dates, timestamps, typos, or images that link directly back to specific Q posts. Sometimes there are deltas, specific posts relating to events exactly on the date, but posted x number of years back.

Every single event, and there have been several each week since the Biden admin came in, has been covered one way or another, nothing seems to be happening by chance. There are too many examples to give but the key message is, there are no such things as coincidences here.

My first example, the most recent to the time of writing, is back to the October 2023 attack on Israel by Hamas – how did the Iron Dome of Israeli intelligence not intercept it? How did they not see this taking place? The attack was on the 7th, but it seems intelligence systems were deactivated a few days before – or not working properly, for some reason.

We were led, by clear comms, to this post, written exactly 5 years ago – no coincidences.

2337 Oct 04, 2018 5:27:07 PM EDT

Q !!mG7VJxZNCl ID: 000000 No. 335

ISRAELI INTELLIGENCE - STAND DOWN.
[TERM_3720x380-2934766692830 01]
Media assets will be removed.
Q

#WWG1WGA   8chan patriotsfight

Unfortunately, as we know, people didn't wake up as quickly as hoped. Q told us to be digital soldiers, that this was the biggest Civilian / Military operation ever and nothing like this had ever happened before - we needed to wake people up to what was happening – largely we failed – but, of course, that was also anticipated.

This means we are headed to a 'Big Scare Event' – and that will be something resembling WWIII.

To get an idea of what and how Q points us towards the film 'The Sum of all Fears' – it's worth a watch if the real one hasn't already happened. As I said, my watch currently makes it five to WWIII.

Example 2: You may have noticed an extra 'L' in a couple of Trump posts on Truth Social, where he 'misspells' the word 'Stolen'.

Here is something to take note of, he never makes any spelling mistakes – not even COVFEFE.

The extra 'L' leads us to this post from 2018

#2478   11/11/18 12:58:18 PM EST Q !!mG7VJxZNCl

Let the unsealing begin.
Let the DEC[L]AS begin.
Let the WORLD witness the TRUTH.
We, the PEOPLE.
JUSTICE UNDER THE LAW.
Q

Remember, Trump will be broadcast live in court expected in March 2024, a case where HE is accused of subverting an election (Ha!) – he can call any witness – he can provide any evidence - the world will be watching!

Just two examples of hundreds – There are no coincidences.

Q is US Military Intelligence; Q tells us Trump is fully insulated by the military despite the Deep State's attempts to remove him.

Go back to the picture, where he is giving his Inauguration speech, who is behind him? – The Military. They gathered behind in a 'we got your back' gesture. But more than that, and this is very important, there are two key personnel with special cap striping. The officer on the Right of the picture with a Gold/Black/Gold striped braid is from The Judge Advocate General branch (think Military Tribunals), and the officer on the left of the picture has braiding with Gold/Blue/Gold - Military Intelligence (enough said).

By the way, it's currently 2023 and Trump is still the Commander in Chief of the USA.

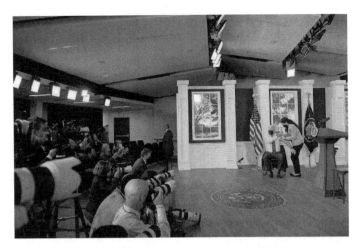

The Big Guy – Joe Biden makes it to the White House.

19. Devolution

They let him steal the diamonds.

What happens when a country is attacked in an act of war by a foreign power? When that power places its dictator puppet in office, and a regime takes over? What happens to the legitimate government, if they are not put in jail, or killed?

Normally, things are drawn up to try and preserve them, like a government in exile, to preserve the nation's security – a Continuation of Government, keeping things as stable as possible until the enemy is defeated. To put this in place, the legitimate Head of State / President / Prime Minister needs to declare an act of war against itself by a foreign power, think Pearl Harbour.

Trump declared two acts of war from foreign adversaries – both mainly China's CCP.

The first was a bioweapon attack – Covid 19.

The second, a cyber-attack – The 2020 election.

Remember, Joe Biden's Inauguration on Jan 20th, 2021, here are some oddities;

1. Biden was sworn in 14 minutes early and before Kamala Harris.

2. Trump leaves on AF1. Biden flies in a small private jet.

3. Cloudy day on the 20th, live inauguration bright and sunny. Reportedly shown in Europe 12 hours early live.

4. Kamala living in some other house other than the VP residence.

5. Bogus CGI extravagant fireworks display that never happened, clearly fake.

6. Senator Roy Blunt with his hands behind his back being escorted out of the Capitol.

7. Pelosi being told not to talk to anyone by some strange woman (with a US Marshal badge) on the 20th.

8. 30k troops for a non-violent virtual inauguration. With 5k there in DC until mid-March, yet no violence to deal with.

9. The White House going pitch black each night with a strange structure being built directly in front of it.

10. Oval office that Biden is signing pretend orders in, completely different from real one.

11. No secret service snipers on the White House roof.

12. No secret service call box on his Bidan's desk.

13. Biden locked out of the White House on the first day.

14. Joe Biden's executive order signatures don't match his actual signature.

15. A 2nd set of nuclear codes left with Trump on his way out.

16. Images of Bill Clinton, Bush, and Obama standing together, Obama glitches and completely disappears for a few seconds.

17. Trump says he'll be back in some form, then files for a new political party several days later.

Why did 'president' Joe Biden receive a shoddy 21-gun salute from Arlington Cemetery, with only 3 cannons, 9-second intervals, with one misfire? – This was protocol for a Military Funeral service!

However, on Wednesday, Jan 20th, 2021, the same day, President Donald Trump received an impeccable 21-gun salute from a battery of 4 cannons (5-second intervals) at Joint Base Andrews in Maryland, just hours before his presidential term ended – this was a perfectly executed Inauguration service!

Also, Dong Jing Wei was the highest-level defector in US history, with trillions of CCP data. The Biden administration, embarrassingly, had no idea he was with the US military – the military didn't tell them. As the Biden motorcade passed, well over half of the military lining the streets turned their backs on him. By the way, anyone seen Trump's motorcade? As of late 2023, it is enormous, 40 odd blacked out vehicles, multiple motorbikes fore and aft, and a heavy-duty ambulance, often with air support – recently Biden was seen carrying his own bags into a taxi – go figure!

Just some things to chew over.

Devolution was a theory proposed by a guy called Patel Patriot (Jon Herold), it was very complex and, I must point out at the time of writing it, he knew nothing of Q, or how it worked, I know this because I heard several interviews with him where I was becoming aware of the parallels, and he seemed not to be. The interviewer thought the same as me, but, on questioning, Jon clearly hadn't delved yet into it.

The Devolution Series involves 25 rather long and complicated essays that would take a month to explain. Although, initially a theory, this has now been proven on many levels, and in several ways.

'Devolution' essentially boils down to a Continuity of Government (COG) Plan in which a sitting President legally and constitutionally transfers the powers of the United States Commander-in-Chief to a group of selected individuals while he is 'removed from power'.

COG ensures that certain red lines are not crossed while the nation is compromised at a governmental level, such as when illegally invaded. As such it protects critical infrastructure and national security at an essential level until a return to power is possible or advantageous, and constitutional.

Key military powers were devised and written into law even before Trump ran for President, in preparation. Namely the Law of War manual and, later, the Military Justice Act. To reiterate, these were introduced specifically to enable 'The Plan'.

To prepare for this military plan, Trump had to put in place several Executive Orders and PEADS (Presidential Emergency Action Documents) giving power to those in charge under certain conditions. COG means remaining in charge, behind the scenes.

Executive Order 13848, was signed on Sept 12th, 2018, declaring a state of emergency in the event of foreign interference in US elections, or covert distribution of propaganda or disinformation - with heavy sanctions.

Executive Order 13959 was signed on Nov 12th, 2020, just after the election which freezes the assets of anyone profiting in dealings with the CCP – with heavy sanctions.

Executive Order 13818 signed December 20, 2017, Blocking the Property of Persons Involved in Serious Human Rights Abuse or Corruption.

There are others that one can easily research, or you can read the whole Devolution series online.

What is very interesting, all the EOs above, including Executive Order 13581 of July 24, 2011, signed by Obama, Blocking Property of Transnational Criminal Organizations, have been repeatedly re-signed by Biden – very strange considering he is likely to fall foul of all of them, so signing his own death warrant. Is it even him???

Don't get me talking about masks again! Certainly, he is being controlled, whoever he is – and by both sides.

Trump is a wartime president, but you can't have two overt presidents, they allowed Biden to appear as the President to show everything that he and his deep state masters are capable of, and just look what they did in just a few years! Wars, lots of them all around the world, the economy crashing, the dollar sinking, the BRICS rising (a good thing), society falling apart – this was set up to show the people exactly what the deep state are bringing. This is their plan, destruction before The Great Reset – You will own nothing.

Meanwhile, COG is in place to stop the crossing of red lines. Trump is the commander-in-chief; he has the military behind him. He is fully insulated as Q tells us and they are bringing the deep state down in the biggest sting operation ever. Does he look rattled? Really?

This is irregular warfare, Information war, moves and counter moves, cloak and dagger, the goodies are the baddies are the goodies, appear weak when strong, appear strong when weak, infiltrate and Psyop. There is no such thing as coincidences, yet they are happening daily. The Khazarian mafia are doomed, in my humble opinion, but they will get very nasty on their way out, no doubt about that.

So, if Trump is in charge and he has the military, why didn't they just storm in and arrest the baddies right away, why did they allow all this hate, death, and misery? That's what everyone says. We thought they would, to be truthful, we were watching Biden's fake inauguration and were expecting to see it happen, it was nail-biting, any time now, any time now, they will strike, perfect opportunity with everyone there. But were they all there? I have seen plenty of footage that seems to be two different days, change of clothing, positions, etc. If it was a legit inauguration gathering, maybe they were going to, and they became aware of a nasty retaliation – a dirty bomb? Maybe Mr Parks was right.

Or maybe they realised anything looking like a spiteful Trump rolling in his ragged army in some kind of a coup, would just not work, and then the deep-state would just survive for another day. The vast majority of people happy to acquiesce – again.

No, the people needed to see exactly how bad the baddies are, let Biden be the Globalist puppet, but let us control him and let's force them into exposing themselves to the point where the people demand an end to their reign, the people must overcome their cognitive dissonance otherwise they will allow a future tyranny. Let us make it all fall apart spectacularly.

Unfortunately, this is a war, a war of good versus evil, God Vs Devil, a final war to end all wars, there will be casualties. It's the only way.

We won't really know how it all plays out - until it all plays out, but I am full of (informed) Hopium.

With all that in mind, it would be interesting to look at Trump's inauguration speech again – I have made discussion notes 'by pen'.

20. The full text of Donald Trump's Inaugural Speech as the 45th president of the United States

"Chief Justice Roberts, President Carter, President Clinton, President Bush, President Obama, fellow Americans and people of the world, thank you.

We, the citizens of America, are now joined in a great national effort to rebuild our country and restore its promise for all of our people. Together we will determine the course of America and the world for many, many years to come. We will face challenges. We will confront hardships, but we will get the job done. Every four years we gather on these steps to carry out the orderly and peaceful transfer of power and we are grateful to President Obama and First Lady Michelle Obama for their gracious aid throughout this transition. They have been magnificent. Thank you.

(Enough of this bullshit, - now listen to this! Note: at this point the Military moves in behind him)

Today's ceremony, however (Yes, however, meaning everything is now different), has very special meaning because, today, we are not merely transferring power from one administration to another or from one party to another, but we are transferring power from Washington, D.C., and giving it back to you, the people. (Hmm, now this is Different! - Military exit, they made their point!)

For too long, a small group in our nation's capital has reaped the rewards of government while the people have born the cost. (The previously mentioned are corrupt cabal mafia - small group an understatement, but yes, the people are bigger, never forget that) Washington flourished, but the people did not share in its wealth. Politicians prospered, but the jobs left and the factories closed. The establishment (Deep State) protected itself, but not the citizens of our country. Their victories have not been your victories. Their triumphs have not been your triumphs and, while they celebrated in our nation's capital, there was little to celebrate for struggling families all across our land.

That all changes starting right here and right now because this moment is your moment. (The military plan is underway) It belongs to you. It belongs to everyone gathered here today and everyone watching all across America. This is your day. This is your celebration, and this, the United States of America, is your country.

What truly matters is not which party controls our government (they are all cabal), but whether our government is controlled by the people. January 20th, 2017, will be remembered as the day the people became the rulers of this nation again. The forgotten men and women of our country will be forgotten no longer.

Everyone is listening to you now. You came by the tens of millions to become part of an historic movement, the likes of which the world has never seen before. (We finally and permanently take down the Khazarian Mafia) At the center of this movement is a crucial conviction that a nation exists to serve its citizens. Americans want great schools for their children, safe neighborhoods for their families, and good jobs for themselves. These are just and reasonable demands of righteous people and a righteous public, but for too many of our citizens, a different reality exists (freedom from tyranny and WEF agendas).

Mothers and children trapped in poverty in our inner cities, rusted out factories scattered like tombstones across the landscape of our nation, an education system flush with cash, but which leaves our young and beautiful students deprived of all knowledge and the crime and the gangs and the drugs that have stolen too many lives and robbed our country of so much unrealized potential. (As purposely planned by the deep-state players) This American carnage stops right here and stops right now. (Maybe it's worth a close look at Hunter's Laptop)

We are one nation and their pain is our pain. Their dreams are our dreams and their success will be our success. We share one heart, one home and one glorious destiny. The oath of office I take today is an oath of allegiance to all Americans. (The corrupt swamp have broken their oaths and are therefore committing treason) For many decades, we've enriched foreign industry at the expense of American industry (treasonous players beholden to the CCP or Ukraine), subsidized the armies of other countries, while allowing for the very sad depletion of our military. (More treason)

We've defended other nations' borders, while refusing to defend our own, (watch what Biden does with the wall) and spent trillions and trillions of dollars overseas, while America's infrastructure has fallen into disrepair and decay. We've made other countries rich while the wealth, strength and confidence of our country has dissipated over the horizon. One by one, the factories shuttered and left our shores with not even a thought about the millions and millions of American workers that were left behind. The wealth of our middle class has been ripped from their homes and then redistributed all across the world. (Watch the

WEF, they want the middle classes destroyed)

But, that is the past (We will drain the swamp) and now we are looking only to the future. We assembled here today, are issuing a new decree to be heard in every city, in every foreign capital, and in every hall of power. From this day forward, a new vision will govern our land. From this day forward, it's going to be only America first. America first. Every decision on trade, on taxes, on immigration, on foreign affairs will be made to benefit American workers and American families. (We declare war with the Globalist Tyrants)

We must protect our borders from the ravages of other countries making our products, stealing our companies and destroying our jobs. Protection will lead to great prosperity and strength. I will fight for you with every breath in my body and I will never, ever let you down. (I know they will accuse me of everything they can think of, impeach me, jail me, try to destroy me. At times, they will seem to defeat me - but I will keep fighting, I will keep strong, and we will win, we planned this for decades - Nothing Can Stop What Is Coming)

America will start winning again. Winning like never before. We will bring back our jobs. We will bring back our borders. We will bring back our wealth. And we will bring back our dreams. We will build new roads and highways and bridges and airports and tunnels and railways all across our wonderful nation. We will get our people off of welfare and back to work rebuilding our country with American hands and American labour. We will follow two simple rules: buy American and hire American. We will seek friendship and goodwill with the nations of the world, but we do so with the understanding that it is the right of all nations to put their own interests first. (We will lead the fight against the globalists and others will follow together we will bring the whole cabal down)

We do not seek to impose our way of life on anyone, (I am and will always be a man of peace, unlike the warmongers before me) but rather to let it shine as an example. We will shine for everyone to follow. We will reinforce old alliances and form new ones (I already have ☺) and unite the civilized world against radical Islamic terrorism, which we will eradicate completely from the face of the earth. At the bedrock of our politics will be a total allegiance to the United States of America and, through our loyalty to our country, we will rediscover our loyalty to each other. When you open your heart to patriotism, there is no room for prejudice. (The patriots will stop the divisions created by the enemy)

The bible tells us how good and pleasant it is when god's people live together in unity. We must speak our minds openly, debate our disagreements honestly, but always pursue solidarity. When America is united, America is totally unstoppable. There should be no fear. We are protected and we will always be protected. (Insulated - don't worry, even when the chips look down, and they will do) We will be protected by the great men and women of our military and law enforcement (Devolution, COG) and most importantly, we will be protected by God. (God wins - Q said)

Finally, we must think big and dream even bigger. In America, we understand that a nation is only living as long as it is striving. We will no longer accept politicians who are all talk and no action constantly complaining, but never doing anything about it (as they are self-serving, installed corrupt puppets). The time for empty talk is over. Now arrives the hour of action. Do not allow anyone to tell you that it cannot be done. No challenge can match the heart and fight and spirit of America. We will not fail. Our country will thrive and prosper again. (Even if we have to have a 4 year pause to expose the cabal)

We stand at the birth of a new millennium ready to unlock the histories of space, to free the earth from the miseries of disease and to harness the energies, industries, and technologies of tomorrow. (My Uncle has Nikola Tesla's drawings, and the cabal bastards hid everything from you - the cure for cancer, unlimited free energy maybe?) A new national pride will lift our sights and heal our divisions. It's time to remember that old wisdom our soldiers will never forget, that whether we are black or brown or white, we all bleed the same red blood of patriots. (Note, they will always accuse us of racism) We all enjoy the same glorious freedoms, and we all salute the same great American flag.

And whether a child is born in the urban sprawl of Detroit or the windswept plains of Nebraska, they look up at the same night sky. They fill their heart with the same dreams, and they are infused with the breath of life by the same almighty creator. So, to all Americans in every city near and far, small and large, from mountain to mountain, from ocean to ocean, hear these words: You will never be ignored again. Your voice, your hopes and your dreams will define our American destiny. And your courage and goodness and love will forever guide us along the way. (NCSWIC to those who dare get in the way)

Together we will make America strong again. We will make

America wealthy again. We will make America proud again. We will make America safe again. And, yes, together, we will make America great again (MAGA). Thank you. God bless you and God bless America. Thank you. God bless America."

Does this sound like the crazy deranged bigot you thought he was? If not, as it shouldn't, maybe you have been cured of your Trump Derangement Syndrome (with a little truth). Truth always rises to the surface, one way or another – like cream. Truth is real and has a permanent energy. Lies require constant propagation, nurturing, feeding, cooperation, and coordination. Lies usually fail in the cover-up, they always fail eventually, someone slips up, someone tries to save their own skin by revealing the guilt of others, it all falls down eventually, the house of cards.

21. Nessun Dorma

"This is the final battle. With you at my side, we will demolish the deep state.

We will expel the warmongers from our government. We will drive out the globalists. We will cast out the Communists, Marxists, and Fascists.

We will throw off the sick political class that hates our country.

We will rout the fake news media and we will liberate America from these villains.

Once and for all."

Donald J Trump.

Here is where I think we are and where we are heading. I may be wrong.

It's positive, maybe I'm just of that disposition. The situation is incredibly fluid, and things are happening at pace, but I have known for a long time that the military and Trump, along with White Hat allies, and the capitulated deep state players (who took a deal) around the world are implementing a plan.

They let Biden win, they let him steal the election. They decided to have a 'pause' or 'break' as Trump and Dan Scavino (a key Q comms source) put it. The only way the masses of blinkered people will wake up to the globalist tyrants is for them to see what they do. The globalists know they have until the 2024 elections to win their war and take control, this makes them desperate and exposed. Their sixteen-year plans concertinaed into four. This was the only way they could be exterminated in full.

Soon after the 2020 election a team of lawyers representing the Trump administration toured the US to deliver basic evidence of election fraud to the state legislatures, I remember watching all with great enthusiasm, they had highly compelling evidence, irrefutable, but mainstream media wouldn't cover it, the main lawyers involved were Rudy Giuliani, Sindey Powell, and Jenna Ellis. Subsequently, all have been hauled into court under threats from the deep state in a case of 'election subversion', (and possibly, they have been 'turned', my hunch is they haven't, even Ellis who is openly criticising Trump on Twitter) – as the radical left do, they reverse the crime back onto the accusers, it's quite a spectacle and they get away with it. Back to the point, Sidney Powell was a military lawyer, and she had such overwhelming evidence involving the Dominion voting machines, that she teased us with her phrase, 'Release the Kraken', it was such damning evidence, with such power, it would devastate any argument the cheating and lying cabal could muster... We waited with excitement for the Kraken to come. Then Powell was suddenly dropped from the team, she seemed to disappear for a few weeks. When she reappeared, she seemed happy to accept her apparent gagging, she seemed very confident and positive, all she said was 'It's going to be BIBLICAL'. She knew something. This was a significant moment for me because I knew that she knew something. Something big. I am convinced she was told of the full plan, to withdraw and let it all play out to its crescendo – which will be of such a scale and so earth-shattering that it can only be described as 'BIBLICAL'. I could see it in her eyes and that was proof enough for me. Recently, they have appeared in court, in an attempt to silence them, they seem to have taken plea deals to stay out of prison, we must always remember the art of war – 'appear weak when you are strong' – they will reappear stronger in the near future, the Kraken will be rereleased – all IMHO of course.

A similar situation happened with Mike Lindell, 'The Pillow Guy', he seemed to have the digital evidence of a cyberattack conducted by China against the 2020 election that successfully switched enough votes in swing states to change the outcome in Biden's favour. We saw this happen in real-time live here in the UK – it was as clear as mud. Dade County, Georgia, votes being switched live, there is never any plausible reason for accumulative votes to go down!

We saw this,

Total votes: Trump 29,391

Total votes: Biden 17,218

Eight minutes later, the next batch comes in, and TaDa!

Total votes: Biden 29,391

Total votes: Trump 17,218

An exact switch of 12,173

Remember Trump asking the Secretary of State for Georgia if he could find some missing votes??? How the hard left twisted that!

The evidence in question is a PCAP (packet capture) file, or files, in which the data sent between computers in China (and other countries) and election equipment in the US. All PCAPs on and around election day was recorded. Naturally, he was discredited by the media. Some of us knew of the PCAP's way before Lindell funded his own expose, we knew of the Italian Leonardo satellite systems and the 'friendly' firefight over the server in Frankfurt.

I think both Lindell and Powell were asked to lay off to allow this period of 'pause' to play out. I firmly believe US military intelligence has all this evidence and it will resurface soon, in court in early 2024, on TV for the world to see, perhaps. Oh, and watermarks are being mentioned of late by DJT, did they? In 2020? That would be an instant Game, Set, and Match. Watch the Water (it's a Q thang)

As soon as they took power, Biden closed their own gas pipeline construction, they left their arsenal of high-grade military equipment in Afghanistan, for the enemy, US soldiers died and US citizens were trapped, Biden did not show any remorse, they stopped building the wall, in fact, they dismantled parts and started to encourage mass illegal immigration, not only the crooks, gang members, and drug cartels from South America, but from the Middle East and China, something like 14 million unchecked (and unvaccinated) illegals ready to cause trouble, create more division, stir up the patriots in an attempt for a civil war and maybe to vote Democrat. Antifa / BLM / Trans and now Jihadi's are all agitated and angry, wound up by their media and the Nazi billionaires who fund them.

Thousands are dying from Fentanyl and hundreds of thousands dropping from their vaccines – People are seeing this.

First came the Russian / Ukrainian war, rather, an incursion by the Russians to take out deep state assets and biolabs. We know the CIA, Graham, McCain, and Newland et al, created a regime change there in 2014 to install their globalist puppet. Money poured into Ukraine and straight back out again into the deep-state players' pockets – the evidence is piling up against the Biden crime family, we saw him bragging about removing prosecutor Shokin, when VP. People know of the sordid stuff on Hunter's laptop and the 52 intelligence top dogs lying about it. 'We The People' are seeing this all play out.

People are seeing the West blow up the Nordstream pipeline, fire missiles into Poland and their media report obvious Propaganda, they are now seeing more credible truth on Twitter (X) and Rumble – but they are also seeing the deep staters desperately trying to close free speech down, setting up their 'Ministries of Truth' – or 'Disinformation laws'. The Twitter files revealed how governments and intelligence services controlled and manipulated groupthink on social media to influence voting.

Everyone is watching the continued push for vaccines, vaccine passports, CBDC's and the desperate climate hoax – they watch the likes of John Kerry talking complete bollocks, how we 'either have farms growing our own food or a planet – we can't have both', he lies. People are seeing Bill Gates buy up farmland and produce MRNA vaccinations in food, people see the stripey skies and feel the chemicals in our atmosphere. Highly suspicious wildfires all over and mass shootings seemingly 'allowed'. Children go missing, Child sex traffickers go to jail, but their customers are ignored. People can see governments ceding their sovereignty to the likes of the WHO and Klaus Schwab's WEF – people can see all the deep state players are working for the WEF and can also see their wealth accumulation. Vaccines, masks, and lockdowns are all looking very nefarious, our politicians didn't abide by their own rules, and it's becoming clear that most didn't even take their poison.

Now we have Palestinians attacking Israel, and, in return, Israel going full blitzkrieg back – instantly we have hundreds of thousands of Hamas supporters on the streets around the world, their numbers boosted by all the illegals each country has welcomed in, housed, fed, and armed (at least with flags – let's see). Trouble is brewing in Iraq and Iran where only three years ago they were all coming together in Trump arranged Middle East peace deals – The Abrahams Accords. China and Taiwan are next up and you can throw a little bit of North Korea in also – it's one massive shit show and all in just three years!

The people can see this.

People can see the kangaroo courts that belong in the 'most fruity' of banana republics, throw everything at Trump, everything, and nothing. People can see this. It's embarrassing. They have the most corrupt people you can imagine, Letitia James, the AG from New York, who has made it her life's ambition to bring down Trump, spending millions on a sham trial, where no crime or victim exists. The judge, Arthur Engoron, is a clown, a buffoon, a narcissist weirdo, who posts topless pictures of himself on high school websites. They made Trump stand for a mug shot, which subsequently boosted his supporters significantly, especially in the black and Hispanic communities – also sold a lot of merch with that brilliant image! Special prosecutor Jack Smith's pathetic case accusing Trump of subverting an election is going to backfire spectacularly. They will try to imprison him in the meantime and that is a possibility, but I do think all is set up for a 2024 election that Trump will win 'bigly'.

As I said before, my watch makes it five to WWIII, or it did, we are now a minute off it.

Trump predicted this a long time ago, and he is also making it clear he can stop it within 24 hours.

He can.

This was all 'allowed' under the safety net of COG (Continuity of Government), The country's key infrastructures are safe. We are, however, at war, there will be casualties.

WWIII is the Big Scare Event that those who know Q, have been expecting.

Things will get nasty and scary, and they need to, the election will happen despite the Black Hats throwing everything against it, they will want it cancelled – Just like Zelinski has cancelled his.

If war doesn't stop the elections, maybe Trump in prison will. If that doesn't work a cyberattack or another virus. Elsewhere, such as Europe, they will increase the cultural divisions, whip up tension on the streets, create false flags to create riots, fuel those riots with antifa, and use the police to unfairly side against the common people. Then blame everything on an imaginary 'Far-Right'. They want civil wars, mass unrest, excuses to suppress liberty with WEF agenda clampdowns.

Yup, they will try everything.

However, ultimately, they won't succeed.

We know from Q posts that 'they caught them all' (3852), there is a 'collection of overwhelming evidence' (4484, 4245), and how they will 'introduce it all legally' (3850), and many more, we knew this a long time ago. He is due to face the trial of the century (and more) in early spring of 2024 – for 'subverting an election', talk about gaslighting - it will be televised, and Trump has the right to equal time to introduce whatever evidence he has – it's called Discovery - and to call whoever to testify (Space Force?). This is the 'Trump Card' mentioned in Q posts (1201, 2936), and increasingly 'comms' are pointing to them. The world will be watching. A different type of 'Discovery Channel'.

Trump has been arrested and had his tax and bank accounts investigated along with those of his family and businesses – setting the precedent for the same to boomerang back on the Obamas, Clintons, and Bidens. This whole pause is one massive sting operation. Think of Hunter Biden and his laptop, he has now been subpoenaed, look at the headlines – 'Hunter becomes the Hunted', this was a Q quote way back in November 2017 - #158, as is often the case, there is a double meaning. In this case, it refers to the deep state hunting down Trump, they have been enticed into a sting operation, they are the hunters who will become the hunted.

I believe the Dems will oust Biden on a '25th' and introduce Michelle Obama, some say 'Big Mike', I've no idea why.

Things are swinging though (genitalia aside), The new speaker of the house, Mike Johnson, minces no words, subpoenas have been issued, The Bidens are being investigated, Homeland Security Secretary Mayorkas, an embarrassment, the subject of many a recent grilling, will be investigated for purposely opening the border to wave in millions of unchecked immigrants (as dictated by the Cabal's agenda, as is widespread in other countries) – and finally(!) a call for investigations and subpoenas regarding the Jeffrey Epstein flights passengers – hopefully a lot of juicy stuff to be documented in this books' follow-up perhaps. Things are so fluid right now, unfurling exponentially. Vivek Ramaswamy - Wow - he just says it all, truth bombs galore, no holding back, a potential DJT VP?? I just hope he has good security. The same needs to be said about the newly victorious Argentinian president, Javier Milei, a more likeable 'Far Right' chap you couldn't wish to meet -a bit hot under the collar though.

In the UK, we have Andrew Bridgen, a lone and very brave MP standing up against the Big Pharma-influenced politicians on both sides, they all rush to leave when he speaks. Easier to blame their ignorance on 'unfortunately not being able to attend' rather than sticking to the ever-more 'wobbly' claim, they are simply following the science. Currently, a sham of a 'Covid inquiry' is taking place, pure theatre, 100% designed to conclude they didn't lockdown hard or quickly enough, 'lessons learnt', yeah sure - they are preparing the eager normies for the next one, whenever the WHO decides it's time.

We Know Your Play-Book. We Can See What You're Up To.

On that note - just a little shout out to the strategists at deep state HQ. You calling us Far-Right all the time is pathetic, anyone speaking out against your totalitarian agendas is much less Far-Right than you are Far-Wrong. 99% of us are mildly 'near centre', libertarians if anything. Tarnishing us with such wildly agitating false labels just typifies your modus operandi. By the way, the 1% are either pond life, or you place them there as agitators.

There are one or two others, and then we have the likes of Laurence Fox, who has been drawn into politics by being brave enough to realise if he doesn't do it, nobody else will. I give him extra praise due to his brilliant portrayal of Hunter Biden in the film 'My Son, Hunter', a film suppressed because it details the sordid contents of the 'laptop from hell', and that was all 'made up Russian disinformation' – everyone knows it wasn't. We have a small group of Euro MEPs speaking out such as Christine Anderson and Mislav Kolakusic, they never get mainstream exposure, but they certainly are becoming more visible, they are incredibly brave, and their messages are getting heard. Having said that we are now watching millions on the streets protesting about the unscrupulous socialist power grab in Spain – the liars and cheats prevail, for now.

The UK, it seems is the head of the snake, but the key battleground is across the pond, if the US falls, the world falls, and if the deep state fails in the US, so does the global house of cards.

The White Hats will prevail, they have installed a 'Ghost in the Machine', a brilliant counter psyop, infiltration works two ways, the enemy has been fooled and drawn into the greatest sting operation ever and they can't backtrack. The 4th Psychological Operations Group, part of US army special operations command describes themselves thus; *'PSYOP Forces are Masters of Influence – the core of information warfare. We conduct influence activities to target psychological vulnerabilities and create or intensify fissures, confusion, and doubt in adversary organizations. We use all available means of dissemination – from sensitive and high tech, to low-tech, to no-tech, and methods from overt, to clandestine, to deception'*. The Ghost Army in WWII- it's worth researching.

The US election will happen, watermarked paper, and voter ID, probably overseen by the military and the world media, and all done in one night. No excuses.

People will be so desperate for peace they will vote for him-'just please make it stop!!'; he alone will be able to reverse the nightmare of WWIII and everything creating it. They will see clear and present nuclear escalation, a thousand times worse than the Cuban Missile Crisis.

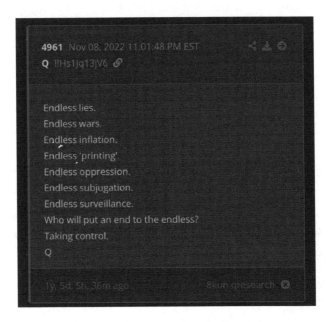

Q also tells us to think of 'Uranium One' (Clintons selling to the enemy – a real treasonous 'Russian Collusion'), Iran, and the film 'The Sum of all Fears' (936,236,199,195 & 194,) a scenario that plays out very quickly with the US getting hit by a nuke, in an attempt to kick off WWIII by blaming Russia but ending with the complete destruction of the Deep State. I don't think a nuke strike will happen, but it may be very close.

Writing this book can be likened to telling the story of a vicious hurricane but completing it before the swirling beast has passed. The hurricane is fluid and unfurling at a rapid rate, it can go anywhere and do anything, all I can do is give my predictions of where it's going, based on what I have at my disposal... ..I trust the real generals and US military intelligence, I see their 'comms'.

The real attack on the deep state will happen at night sometime in November 2024 – by vote - and in the morning God Wins.

We are in a clown world, it is a nightmare, how do we get home? It's as simple as clicking our heels three times. The people need their hearts, their brains, and courage.

Like changing the rule allowing a VP to disallow the results of an election, they shot themselves in the foot – they get steered into these mistakes by the White Hats. They will play very dirty, things will become very scary, but the hunter will become the hunted.

'The Sum of all Fears' features Nessun Dorma, gloriously sung by Pavarotti, a soundtrack as the deep state players are slain and ruthlessly taken out.

It starts with this line:

Nessun dorma! **Nobody shall sleep!**

And ends with this:

All'alba vincerò! Vincerò!, vincerò! **At dawn, I will win! I will win! I will win!**

Release the Kraken

It's Going To Be Biblical

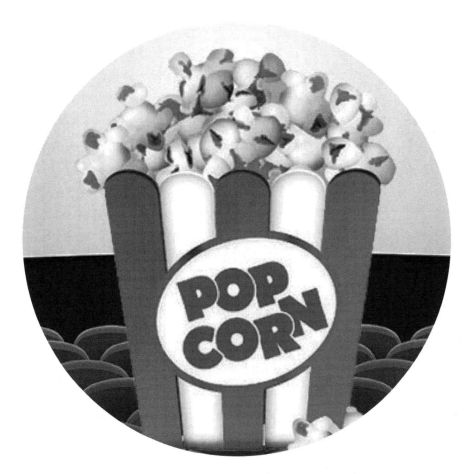

Nothing Can Stop What Is Coming

Printed in Great Britain
by Amazon

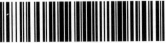

35654616R00141